A startling and lovely configuration of stories, endlessly echoing and reverberating, haunted and haunting. Gretchen E. Henderson creates a sublime and mysterious music all her own.

~ Carole Maso, author of *Mother and Child* and *Ava*

The House Enters the Street is beautifully written, confident and complex. I was appreciative of its language and intelligence, mindfulness and scope.

~ Rikki Ducornet, author of *Netsuke* and *Phosphor in Dreamland*

Intricate and complex, but never confusing, this dazzling novel is as eloquent as it is original. As if content and form were singing in rounds, Gretchen E. Henderson's vibrant characters—their voices and their stories—emerge with careful intent and true beauty to achieve what reads as almost miraculous.

~ Binnie Kirshenbaum, author of *An Almost Perfect Moment* and *The Scenic Route*

... a frenetic "love story" that sound[s] more like every beautiful idea that could be thought of while walking through a city street on childhood, philosophy, history, and yes, love.

~ Stephen Thomas, writing for *The Millions*

THE HOUSE ENTERS THE STREET

(NOVEL)

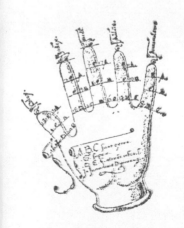

GRETCHEN E. HENDERSON

STARCHERONE BOOKS • BUFFALO, NY

General Editor: Ted Pelton
Book Editor: Rebecca Maslen
Cover Design: Claudia Esslinger
Proofreaders: Brian Mihok and David Neth

Library of Congress Cataloging-in-Publication Data

Henderson, Gretchen E.
The house enters the street / Gretchen Henderson.
  ISBN 978-0-9837405-1-3 (pbk.)
  1. Scandinavians--Iowa--Fiction. 2. Immigrants--Fiction.
  3. Photographers--Fiction. 4. Families--California--Fiction.
  5. Domestic fiction. 6. Experimental fiction. I. Title.
  PS3608.E52595H68 2012
  813'.6--dc23
  2012022961

State of the Arts

NYSCA

This book is made possible with public funds from the New
York State Council on the Arts, a state agency.

for Ethan,
always & all ways

Their clothes too were coarse and shabby.... Straightway they took sharp knives and began to rip up some of the seams and welts...which had all been stitched up in those dresses in so artful a fashion that nobody could have suggested the fact. For when they took leave of the Great Can they had changed all of the wealth that he had bestowed upon them into this mass of rubies, emeralds, and other jewels, being well aware of the impossibility of carrying with them so great an amount in gold over a journey of such extreme length and difficulty. Now this exhibition of such a huge treasure of jewels and precious stones, all tumbled out upon the table, threw the guests into fresh amazement, insomuch that they seemed quite bewildered and dumbfounded.

~ Ramusio, *Collection of Voyages and Travels: Book of Marco Polo*

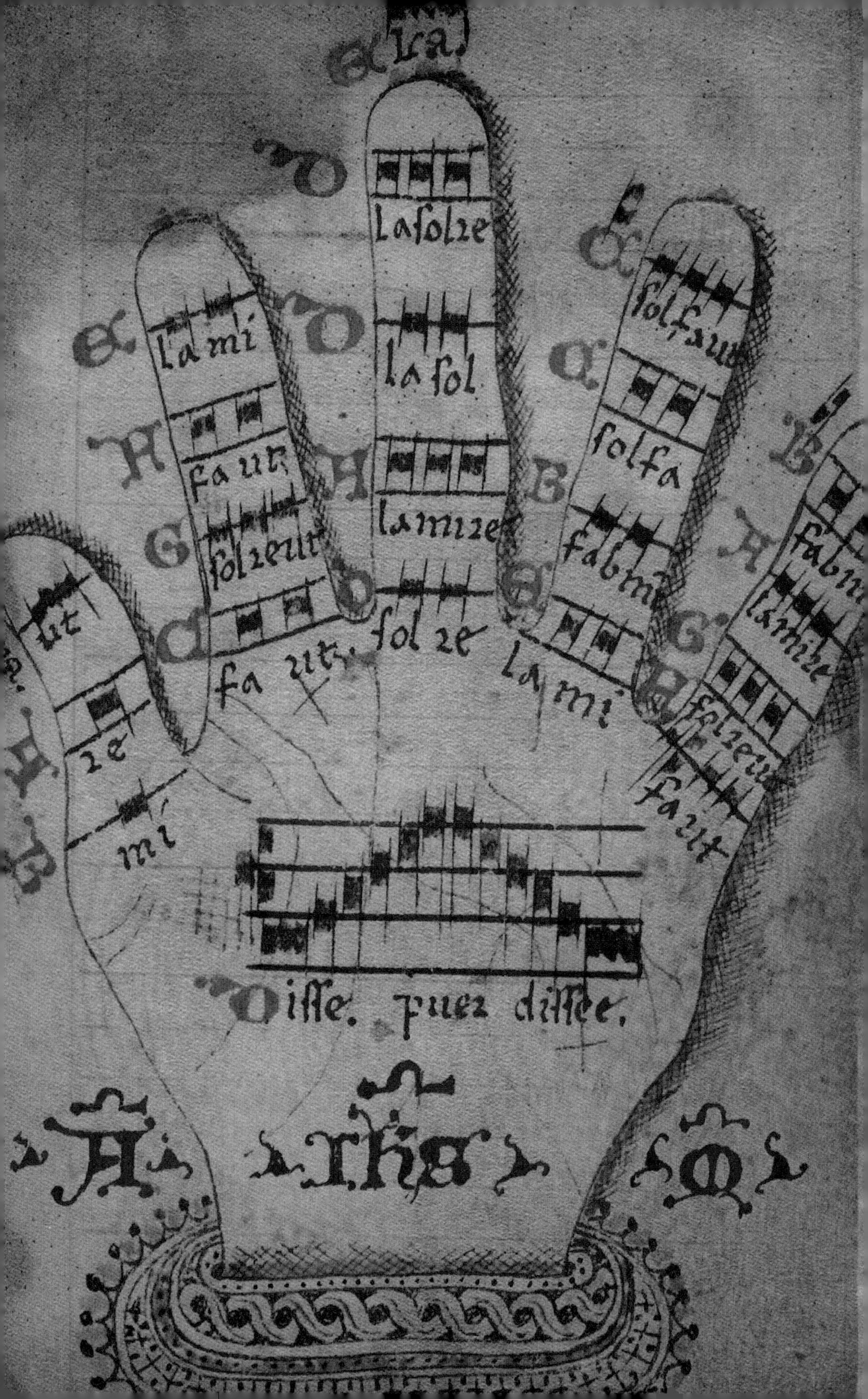
la
la sol re
la sol
la mi re
sol re
la mi
fa ut
sol re ut
fa ut
ut
re
mi
sol fa ut
sol fa
fa b mi
la mi
fa b mi
la mi re
sol re ut
fa ut
Disse. puer disse.
Ihs

MODULATIONS*

i. *Famuli tuorum* (red)
ii. *Ut queant laxis* (orange)
iii. *Solve polluti* (yellow)
iv. *Resonare fibris* (green)
v. *Labii reatum* (blue)
vi. *Mira gestorum* (indigo)
vii. *Sancte Joannes* (violet)

(* Translation available on page 128, colored by the Coda on page 209.)

I

We share her view and multifold sensations, as the interior literally takes in the surrounding exterior buildings and activities....and the numerous laborers are dispersed widely and forward. Houses surge into the foreground. Windows multiply across the facades of fragmented buildings....'The Street Enters the House' refers to the house of the construction site and to the larger social dimension of urban expansion, both of which compel the privacy and domesticity of the interior sanctum to confront the public interactions and boisterousness of the world outside.

(from *Boccioni's Materia*)

Famuli tuorum

Go to the cupboard at waist height, where you keep staple ingredients, and retrieve a Campbell's can. Flavor doesn't matter – there, *Condensed Tomato*. Take care when reaching, since you're not supposed to extend too high or too low. Your muscles don't work the way normal muscles do. Bring the can to the electric opener; secure the top under the magnetic arm. As the opener grinds the metal edge, tomato stench escapes. Your hands appreciate reclusion; you can't use a manual opener for the same reason that you can't grip a knife to cut tomatoes. Remove the can as steadily as possible, or red paste will drip down the label. Don't worry about dabbing goop off the cherubic children; pour the can's contents into a saucepan; your task is almost complete. The soup is condensed, so fill the empty can with water to add before turning on the gas.

With the burner flaming, tomato scent spreads. You are growing partial to the flavor; for too long you were accustomed to homemade soups and stews thick with chunks of potatoes, carrots, and other spearable and scoopable ingredients. Your new criterion is sippability. Thin soups – bouillons and broths – can be served in the belly of a mug. Your special spoon, fork, and knife with thick rubber handles help you relearn to hold, cutlery and otherwise. As you are relearning to sit, to stand, to breathe, to touch, to write with a pen, between your index and middle fingers. That task is especially difficult because it is more than a physical act; it enables your communication. Your handwriting is slowly improving, although you still can't type, cut, grip, play piano, or perform tasks that make the pain return too quickly: prickling inside your fingers, stabbing in your wrist, as muscles in your back contract out-of-control. You stand crooked and humpbacked. Your hands collapse to flat or clamp into claws, disabling their use.

Months earlier, a team of reputed neurologists and physical therapists in California recommended that you sacrifice your place in a piano performance program. "What you love may cripple you," they said. "You have to choose, for your life." By that time, you had already lost so much – the ability to play, teach, perform, write, drive, grasp, sit and stand, your independence – but were afraid to withdraw, in case you might never get back on track. Another patient, a former flautist from the Sydney Symphony, told you that she had given up her career, relocating to the States, and after two years was still rehabilitating: practicing diaphragmatic *breathing* (you say the word again and again to your voice-activated word processor, which miswrites *grieving, grieving*), reconciling herself to exorbitant debt from medical bills, and planning a different vocation. "The best thing for you to do," a physical therapist advised you, "is to try soft, not hard." He added, "Your body has too high a tolerance for pain."

The medical team committed you to an intensified program in an attempt to improve you in condensed time. Trying to revive one sense, they blocked another. Beside paralyzed stroke patients and amputees with reconstructed appendages – each following different recovery protocols – you began: learning Braille with closed eyes, matching plastic Fisher-Price Oreos around differently-shaped rubber creams, and pairing miniature figurines, safety pins and barrettes, hidden in a box among dry rice and barley. You walked blindfolded to navigate through your fingertips. To regain a normal sense of touch. Clenching a fist under your chin, you used your other hand to support your elbow, making a pyramid (because a triangle is the most stable of shapes), putting your neck in temporary traction – a position the PT team called "The Thinker." You constantly became "The Thinker," whenever you sneezed and when you sat, to keep your neck stabilized. Your family joked about it, since you had to move back home; your two sisters tried to make you laugh, to see you smile again. Your long hair got cropped, short as a boy's. Your inventory continued to grow: the Braille book, children's toys, supportive back pads, a neckbrace, halved rubber balls to wrap inside your palms to remind them to arch, an air pillow and styrofoam cylinders on which to exercise your spine, voice-activated computer equipment, a reading stand, a dictaphone to tape-record notes to remind you what to do, and Leukotape to bind your head, neck, back, wrists and fingers, for your body to remember where its parts connected.

 Your physical therapists gave you a patient handbook to explain the science behind the sensitivity: "This may represent a type of negative learning where there is a disorganization of the representation of the hand on the cortex of the brain. If the sensory representation of the hand is seriously disorganized and degraded, coordinated fine motor movements can deteriorate efficiency and accuracy. In some cases the hand may act like it has a life of its own when performing a certain target task."

You've watched your new, loose handwriting improve between sensory trials of touching and gripping, before trying target tasks that make the pain return too quickly, so your body metamorphoses and makes you humpbacked, with useless hands.

You withhold and wait. To try again.

Again and again.

Your condition didn't happen overnight, your physical therapists say. It's been building for years and may take as long to reverse, if possible.

After getting back some mobility, you take out more loans and move cross-country (with help to travel) to recover what you can, on your own, where no one will compare who-you-were to who-you-are becoming.

In your small apartment, shared with strangers, you close your bedroom door not to be seen supine on your spine rolls or wrapped in your neck brace, so no one will fuss or perceive less than your abilities, or know that you have never tried harder – softer – for anything in your life.

You renew lessons in singing because a scholarship provides them for free, and singing proves a test: a body can't make sufficient sounds without proper posture and support, without tension. You try to breathe in the new way that you've been taught, to relax, to sing. To rest and distract your hands.

You've watched your hands attempt movements, as physical therapists encouraged you to observe and imitate healthy hands. You grow easily humiliated and jealous of the arch of other palms, the ease of opposable thumbs, and facilities to grip, cut, and sew. Hearing a piano played, you sense your fingers wanting to move, former motions that they can no longer negotiate. You can't play music, or paint, sculpt, photograph, or handwrite. Before you took for granted an appendage that over time has been used for more than grasping – for foretelling the future through palmistry, for healing with gestures called mudras, for communicating through sign language, for teaching sight-singing syllables to medieval choir boys, when books were truly *manu*-scripts, illuminated by hand. "When you get better, this will be something to write about," a friend suggests when the final tests for degeneration return negative. You're relieved by the news but feel a kind of revulsion when she says that, as if it were worthwhile to lose so much – your ability to make music, to communicate in the most personal way you know how – and you still have a long recovery ahead of you. Besides, writing aggravates symptoms since it uses the same micro-muscles that were used to play piano. You merely nod at her, slightly, because your neck is stiff and you don't want to waste energy on disagreement.

Finding physical relief from exercising on spine rolls, frequent walking, moving in a pool, Tai Chi and Qi Gong, your body learns new ways to negotiate space. Your Master's degree is the least of your worries, as you learn to reeducate your body. Day after day, week after week, semester after semester, you start to trust yourself again. With a new boost of confidence, you study part-time job descriptions (line by line before applying, because you've never quit anything in your life) to break out of your cocoon, into the world, without setting yourself back. You are deep in debt, aching to work. You find what seems the right job, related to music, albeit administratively. Bringing your new flat keyboard (nicknamed "no force," an electronic godsend), you quash shame and dismiss your boss's raised brows with a smile and a casual comment, that the keyboard is merely ergonomic. She ignores the job description and sends you off to do her personal shopping to decorate her office, lifting and hammering, as well as tasks of another assistant who is yet to be hired, which puts your body in jeopardy to the point that you have to explain your reason for quitting, as politely as you can, which is followed by her chastisement (although you never said the word and refuse to be labeled), "Are you telling me that you're *dis-abled*?," followed by a stream of insults that are condescending and short-sighted, but you don't care, just want to stop hurting, even to cut off your hands, so everyone will see visibly what you lack. So you won't have to avoid situations (like eating with other people, because someone inevitably seems to comment on your silly-looking silverware) or explain anything, ever. Since when you manage your condition, you look more or less "normal" (whatever "normal" means).

Under artificially-lit constellations at Grand Central Station, as trains arrive and depart, you walk back to the subway and watch commuters, knowing any of them may carry something invisible but remain silent, for fear of being judged. As your train rattles and twists, you stand without gripping a pole, feet spread to balance, and continue thinking ("The Thinker," after all) about what people lose, about what empties and fulfills a person, about how we all turn out in the end. You feel like an entirely different person and wonder where life is leading. Although doctors aren't sure how or if you'll fully recover, they keep encouraging different methods to retrain your body to remember what it's supposed to know. And you keep hope, even when discouraged, wanting to be independent, to feel that glee of not worrying about physical obstacles, to know the security of good health. You recall moment after moment, what you've experienced or imagined (everything blurs), including a young woman (was that *you?*, questioning so much about yourself now) embarking with a human rights delegation for a war-wracked country in Central America. As you sat in the plane, tears matted your cheeks, and a companion expressed concern. You responded, "I'm not crying from sadness. I'm just saying goodbye to my old self."

You want to say goodbye, again, to your old self. As if your self should be the center of your story –

Deliberating which way to go, you stop by the Met because, in winter, it's frigid and harder to walk outdoors for long stretches. The Met is snug and bustling, and since your student body card allows free admittance, you treat the museum as your gym, with labyrinthine galleries like an asymmetrical track, only better, because delights emerge with every turn. You circle, again and again, sometimes without stopping, other times taking breaks, distracting your hands by scrutinizing shapes and shades of paintings, sculptures, stained glass, mosaics, marquetry, *wunderkammern*, carpets, mummies, and ancient statuary without heads, arms, or hands. Museum-goers revere the statues for their partiality, which makes you watch people as part of the art, until skylights above the Temple of Dendur darken with dusk.

On the verge of leaving, the museum's shop beckons you to see a book, open to *The Street Enters the House*, exploding with colored planes, folding and unfolding, vibrantly moving in stillness.

Step by step, you leave the museum, warmed by thoughts

of the painting, by art's animation that colors the cold, as you walk back to your small room: your temporary home.

Your friend suggests again, "You should write about this."

You consider the idea, now that you sense progress and can stand without your head unbearably top-heavy, now that you don't feel like you're moving through mud and can hold a book, sit to listen to a performance, even if you can't play piano or type on a regular keyboard without regressing, without reawakening symptoms. Even if you can't make music in the way you once knew, at least you can voice-activate words – trying to make a new kind of music – listening while walking through museums or to the grocers, where you find a can of Campbell's *Alphabet Soup*, which you haven't eaten in years.

It boils in a saucepan. Turn off the heat, and let it cool. While you're waiting, read and rearrange letters: *B, E, A, D, G, C, F,* and the rest. Since the road to recovery isn't straight, you can't spell this out, write about it directly, or physically write it at all. You think of it as happening to someone else, or a tale where a body forgets to be a body and hides its heart in a tree, or a legend where someone cannot speak and puts stones in her mouth to learn to articulate. Or a story that stops and starts, stops and restarts, modulating, because the end keeps changing. Like you've improved and deteriorated, again and again. But because or in spite of the end or the beginning, you've learned to relish this moment in the middle. And at least, you can speak. You fall asleep, reimagining the story and how to tell it, *in medias res,* beginning with the young woman who wasn't crying from sadness, beginning with *her,* the one saying goodbye to her old self, the one who's going home:

Ut queant laxis

She's going home. Not straight away, crow dart-of-a-black-arrow going home, but a curvaceous, loopy, round-about, colorful waving (good-bye, hello, good-) course of going home, not by plane, train, coach or car, but by foot through labyrinthine halls and echoing galleries, where marble athletes lack legs, hands, noses (breathing); floor-to-ceiling canvases, blue nudes & strung guitars, head-dressed gazelles with locked horns, beaded earflaps, iron mudfish in pendant masks (breathing). Like a whorled conch, murmuring: voyeurs whisper, stare and bend to listen (knees crack, she hears, shuffling and *Look!*) to incisions and scars – what doesn't speak is broken (between each line & curve) echoes:

This is what happens when there is space & time & hope, she thinks, listening while walking among pedestals & glass cases with palmette finials, rearing maned horses, carved paws on lotus leaves beside bronze belly guards ("Aisonidas, the son of Kloridios, took this"), dolphin-riding *hoplites* ("foot soldiers"), flute players, incised choruses, bronze & terracotta sphinxes perched on horizontal flanges, *greaves* ("shin guards") & spears & water jars & *kernos* ("the receptacles probably contained foodstuffs of various kinds, perhaps also flowers"), pomegranates on oil lamps, *stelae* depicting ravens & a leaping white fox, an omen to decipher, as it races down a horse's back on an architectural frieze between a colonnade & funerary monument, with two lines of dactylic hexameter, expressing grief over death in a pattern called *boustrophedon* ("ox-turning") because the text turns at the end of each line, right to left in alteration, as oxen turn a plough at each furrow's end, zigzagging like she coils through echoing galleries & labyrinthine halls, among pedestals and glass cases – she: the one among statues and foreign tongues, the one who's going home:

But it's not as easy as that. Home is where the heart is, so the saying goes, and though hers beats somewhere inside this cavity, tangled muscles and twisting bones have made it hard for the pulse to be heard, while she tries to move in dreams over mountains, fording streams & oceans to sail to new ports. She feels history on her back like a weight, but a load that needs to be borne, over mountains & rivers & oceans, like the dream of an old barefoot man with a sac-cloth of apple seeds, who thought the world would be better when branches tangled toward sun & grew fruit – like she believes, if she takes seeds (not knowing even which kind they are), if she scatters them across the earth, the old myth may come to life again, once upon a time, ever after – if she reaches out her hand to yours, and you take what she offers and swallow seeds, a tree will grow inside you, and you will bear fruit.

Solve polluti

It was all about the fruits of labors, not only on land: at sea. Faar's life began at sea. Waves rolled outside his window, where he watched watery horizons. His father had disappeared on a voyage to *terra incognita*, where horned narwhales swam under ice, where profit lulled into frozen floes. The young Faar began to dream of cloud lagoons, bellied sails, and wind. The wayfaring trait had been inherited. He decided to wander.

Cousins on the other side of the world sent him a letter to marry their eldest daughter: *S-v-a-n H-a-r-d-t. I-o-w-a*, they wrote, without mentioning the distance between bordering seas. Faar assumed oceans existed near their home. He was young, then. By ship, he departed with dried apple seeds, an overcoat, compass, and words: *fjords, bøndegard, fisker.* Heading toward Hardts, he arrived ashore and rode a box that made its own clouds. Smokestacks puffed from tracks that led to black barren soil, where land spread, gaunt and gleaned.

It was April. The Hardt's wooden barn jutted against a flat farm and overgrown sky: a first sight that made the young man lonely. He felt anchored between one ocean and another, moored, because his new family lived land-locked. They did not feel the pull of tides.

Or so he guessed. It was barely spring. He married the girl from the letter: *Svan. Svan e Lars Röne.* Seeds were planted in earth and watered for growth. Rains came, thundering. Days after storms, sun rifled tufts to make fields glimmer like oceans. Stalks drowned in rows. The barn's body hid, with its roof sailing like an upside-down skiff.

Slowly, Faar grew to love his inland sea. Liquid layers seeped into his dreams and yielded new sights Faar had not imagined. At harvest, he shucked closed ears. The land was deheaded and foddered, and new tides advanced. White, heavy drifts whirled and moaned; snow packs coiled in frozen crests. Other winds carried fresh-fall like foam, like white spiders flung to the wind, unfurling blanched gossamer strands. Flakes met drifts and covered everything: the fields, barn, trees whose branches stretched bare, then budded, above snowdrops and crocuses. Movements continued, all four seasons, after he reaped roots for Svan so she grew into *Mor:* with the birth of their *datters.*

There were three *datters:* Eva, Una, Holde. Three in one, one in three. Born the same day. The year was 1910. Before the girls knew words were w-o-r-d-s, Faar cradled them and chanted language that grew from *fjords* and *fisker, krapp sjø* and *tun sjø –* choppy, short waves; hard, heavy water. He described drawings on cave walls: ships and Ymir, Odin, Thor. He told of trolls, elves, giants, *vetter, draugens,* sprites who swam in the sea, and witches who dressed as insects and held possessions to make owners victims. The Giant who Had No Heart in His Body hid his separated soul in common objects: an egg, a duck, a well, an island, a far-off lake.

When the triplets grew to realize losses could be found, they sought hidden bits of the Giant's heart – estranged in tree stumps, jars, nests, and ponds. More than blood and bones, Faar's stories made the *datters* realize their watery composition, which could pulse *this* or *that* to the surface, or bear things away, in this new-found sea.

Losses were always waiting to be found: buried under de-headed corn stalks, stored in the cellar with Mor's preserves, nested in knotholes of trees whose roots suckled groundwater. Roots rerouted the girls, as stories transformed their senses: sights into sounds, touches into smells, tastes into colors. In summer's heat-blazed roads, mirages revealed liquid horizons and conjured the taste of tears. New senses ripened with each new connection: *this* with *that*; *here* to *there*; *before* with *after*. *Life* with *death*.

The girls were born on the same day, same year. That suggested a pattern. But everything didn't follow the same course. Holde, the third of the three, died at four years. She tried to comfort a rabid fox in a corncrib, and its teethmarks led her to follow its fits and foaming. The family had no Forget-me-nots (bright blue or white, arranged in a curving spike; a remedy against serpent bites, syphilis, and mad dogs) to feed her dying mind. Her shroud was a little black frock, tucked in a tight pine box built by Faar. She died in winter, and her body remained in a corner of the barn by the stenched pigpen, until the ground thawed and spring popped through snow.

To the remaining sisters, the loss of their likeness was the loss of part of themselves. They had been one in three, three in one, and could exist only in proportion. The triplets became twins to those who observed them, in name only, because their dead sister split her spirit between them. How else could everything be explained? Holde hid the rest of herself in tree stumps, jars, nests, and bones.

Resonare fibris

Years later, Avra flew over a valley that appeared like a hand. The sight was familiar but foreign. Fingerish peaks reached skyward, above knuckled crests, bearing snow runoff to the valley's palm. A sleepy town pocked the west bank of the river, molten at sunset, veined with tributaries. Ridges stretched to shadow. In dusky meadows, lone houses sparked like fireflies, as glass windows and metal roofing caught lingering slants of sun, full moonlight; then earth appeared to vibrate, as if it were alive – as if it might shake those who stood on solid ground, who were slowly awakening to learn that nothing is secure as it appears to be.

Avra remembered having been there, to visit her grandmother, after her mother died. Her grandmother had introduced herself with a divining rod. From the cab of a cobalt campervan, the old woman called herself Eva and said that her stick led to water, at least to ground above untapped wells. "If someone chooses not to dig, not to wish, that's another matter entirely," Eva said. "All wells are for wishing." While the engine rumbled, Eva also procured a homemade birdhouse, crafted from recovered trash, likening herself to a jackdaw who pecked among ruins to build a nest. Eva was a local collector then, when Avra was ten and learned that her grandmother was alive, not dead like her mother, but living like a hermit peddling notions and knickknacks. That was the first summer they spent together. Avra flew from her father's home in Memphis to Portland, took a bus over the mountains, and met Eva in the campervan at a roadside stop.

They went to a triangular house, an A-frame. It hid high up the canyon, deep in the forest beside a stream. The structure brimmed with specimens from Eva's collection: a pink soapstone face with enlarged eyes, an old clawfoot bathtub filled with rusting license plates, a plastic Buddha that could be plugged in a socket to light up his lotus. No niche was unfilled. Vines and herbs filled seams of walls, under timbers lined with shells, fossils, snake molts, feathers, bones and speckled eggs, on a granite foundation that glinted with crystallized quartz.

It was impossible to sit without touching. Walking around, with tempted fingers, Avra didn't know what to think of it all – particularly her grandmother, who peeled off dog fennel near the baseboard and pressed it to Avra's nose to smell. Eva explained that herbs of all sorts were sewed, knotted, woven, hammered, even glued into walls, like a Turkish carpetmaker or Amish quilter hides history in stitches, shapes, patterns. "Can you make something of this?" she said, pressing Avra's hand to fronds. Eva wouldn't prepare tinctures or antidotes from roots or leaves, or cultivate raw specimens – "let them be what they will" – but sought materials with latent curative properties to incorporate into her home. "Something will happen, as for what, we'll wait and see," she explained to her granddaughter, whose back was pressed to the wall with bated breath, trying not to smell fennel, reputed to ward off *ma-lar-ia* (whose name derived from "bad air" before its cause was clear, Eva said), as Avra wished that the divining rod might zap her a well to China or somewhere else far, where she wouldn't be stewed by this witch. And after Avra pressed so hard against the wall that she paled and fainted, Eva brushed hair out of her eyes and sang something wordless, remembering only the tune.

"She has an active imagination," Avra's teacher told her father that fall, when she returned to Memphis and was assigned to write an essay about her summer.

But it turned out that Eva was neither witch nor conjurer, nor did her broomstick do anything but sweep. The day after Avra arrived, they began preparations. Eva didn't account for Avra's age and gave her articles about seasonal specimens and growth regions, with words like *deciduous* and *angiosperm*, while outfitting the campervan with supplies: maps, plant guides, homemade drying racks, and notebooks for recording inventory. It was a system to be honed through each successive summer. Avra learned Latin classifications and common names: *Genus species*, followed by an initial to indicate the "discoverer" (*L* for Linneaeus), categorizing and cross-referencing, diagramming flowering shrubs and sketching root systems, noting growth conditions – winter dormancy and spring budbreak – all to take into consideration for planning the route of that season's trip.

"Where did you come from?" Avra asked, shortly before their first departure, noticing a carved sign that read, *Here all dwell free.*

"Here. There's no there."

"Where?"

Eva didn't respond. Avra withheld further questions.

Trips led them far from the valley. Summer after summer, for five years, they camped near the Graveyard of the Pacific, near jagged-ridged Sawtooths and Bitterroots, geysers and bubbling mudpots, parched arroyos of Badlands and the Great Plains, spreading away from rank-upon-rank of ever-extending Rockies. Depending on the year's precipitation and sought specimens, trips branched past the Yukon to Denali, banked in fog or sunlit in the middle of nights. Their southernmost route bypassed coral-colored Arches toward the Garden of the Gods, Painted Desert and Four Corners, where Avra put each of her hands and feet in a different State. All the trips revolved around collecting herbs and planting apple seeds.

Revisiting half-a-decade of buried memories, Avra noticed the charred divining rod. The garage hadn't burned. It was as strange a structure as the A-frame. Modeled on a Yupik cache and accessed by a hand-built ladder, it had served as a storage house, organized and wired by guidance from *Black and Decker* manuals. They had stored maps and supplies in cubbies, now empty, except for a few books and wall hangings. "Something will happen, as for what, we'll wait and see," Avra heard her dead grandmother's voice again, as she recalled features on antiquated maps: an imaginary race of headless men with faces on chests, dragons with blossoming tails and a literally-red sea; camels near horseback-riders beside text adapted from Marco Polo's accounts and, off the Indian coast, pearl divers. "At some point in time, every corner of *terra* is unknown to one person and home to another. You'll have to chart your own *incognita*."

It was spring, then summer. Seasons were fusing. The transience gave Avra comfort, rerooted her in the cycle of time, merging between years and decades, since she lived outside all of them. Smoke filled her nostrils; then it was raining and she smelled sweet rot of apples. In the orchard, she wasn't wet. No footprints followed her spectral body. She viewed the world without eyes, heard without ears and tasted, smelled, and touched without a mouth, nose, hands.

The clouds parted. Sun shone. In the dirt lay scraps of waterlogged paper, smeared almost beyond legibility. Piecing together phrases end to end, she glanced a question before letters scattered like birds, as she walked outward in spirals, simulating what she'd once learned in a wilderness rescue course – in case a member of the group went missing. Round and round the house, in ever-widening circles, she searched for more remains by trudging without feet, moving through air thick as mud, weighted by senses and sounds that someone alive in the forest might have perceived only as whirs of wind. No trees fell but she heard them creakily grow.

It was raining again, and something flailed in Avra's throat. Inside the carport, she glimpsed a sketch on the wall:

the skeletal A-frame, webbed with lines from doors, windows and foundation corners, to a vanishing point – without yard or sky, floating among diagonals like marionette strings. The house, pulled in all directions. She thought of it as a map, made by explorers who neglected details and didn't leave a key, or who purposefully disproportioned features with two northward arrows to throw a navigator off course. Small spirals of smoke curled from the surface, from the chimney and unmarked vents. Then the paper flamed, curled orange into black, fell as a pile of ash, and left her alone, not knowing where to go.

Famuli tuorum

You've entered the house – of mirrors – warped like a funhouse, labeled *La casa entra nella strada*, a painting in place of a wooden sign carved *T-u-s-s-e-b-o*, "House of the Crazies." This house in this forest (lacking a Buddha whose lotus alights) holds two bedrooms and a bath, with faucets and a sump pump that overflows, a wood-burning stove and kitchen where you make *rosetter, krumkake, fattigmand,* and *sandbakkels* with your petite grandmother, who rarely sits still. There's always something to do. Cooking, vacuuming, adopting foster children, playing practical jokes on your grandfather, she loves laughter. During the Depression, she supported her family when her father was ill by standing in a department store window for hours brushing her teeth; now she dyes her still-brunette hair gray, so her friends won't feel bad. Without her daughter (an aunt who you never met), she and your grandfather care for you in summers.

In the living room, clay pipes line ceiling rafters above a brick fireplace, flanked by a woodpile, carved duck decoys, and basket of *Midwest Living*. Closets and a hutch hold fishing poles, an old metal communion cup hewn in the South Seas during World War II, a spinning wheel and copper teakettle that traveled by Scandinavian ship, carvings from East Africa and books about Human Ecology, *On Death and Dying*. Russian choral music rumbles from speakers among stitched *hardanger* and hundreds of butterpats glued to the wall in the shape of a diamond. The house is filled with laughter, despite ghosts (the daughter dead of cancer at 27) because your grandparents believe in grace, in mystery, and in the sacrament of black coffee. At the top of the stairs, a wall hosts black-and-white photographs; you've not met most people who stare from the frames but can tell hundreds of stories about them; their lives feel as real as your own. Your family's myth keeps you moving, animated, even when you leave the forest to return to the city. You know your place in these stories. You rarely look in a mirror, not needing it to remind you who you are.

In that house, apart from laughter, there's always the undermurmur of the river. Trees bend in wind, cracking. Stars whisper like conches, if only you could reach to the sky and pull one down to your ear. In the dirt, you find chips of blue and white china and a broken gold pocketwatch (with an inscription you can't read, except the year: 1910). On that lane, your younger sisters are baptized, and the three of you run through woods, wild little women, cross-country skiing, swimming, planting zinnias, cutting peonies, toting buckets of snap peas and raspberries (at least, those that aren't eaten straight off the vine), being licked by a lapful of Pointer puppies and laughing, watching snowflakes glow by moonlight in winter, silently, after everyone else falls asleep. Down by the river, in summer, you catch your first fish and retreat there alone, to listen to voices of grandparents, parents, and sisters drift down from the house. They call and coax you to return, to sing. Back home, in choir, you are called "the little giraffe" since your voice seems too big for your gangly body. Here you prefer to sing by the river, where wind carries sounds downstream, where only the forest hears.

At night, the river continues to murmur. Long after everyone goes to bed, lamps stay lit low. You sit alone with your grandfather, a retired pastor with a heart condition, full-bellied with white hair as frenzied as Einstein's. He fusses with telescope parts, around scattered books and old records, which by dawn will be set back in place by your grandmother. You and he whisper about black-and-white photographs, half-a-century old. He removes them from worn boxes. The ribbed edges of prints from Brownie cameras fill booklets, small as the size of your palms. He shuffles through small and enlarged prints: of a Chippewa chieftess named Sagawagesheguk (he remembers names as if they were his own; not knowing how to spell them later you sound out remembered syllables, *Sagawa...*) so grand that she needed two full-grown men to help her move. She taught him the meaning of *gesis* (with a glottal *g*, long *e*, soft *i*). When her tribe trekked to a lake and sat for hours repeating *gesis, gesis, gesis*, he didn't understand until they returned to camp, and she told him that they'd gone to witness the rising of *the moon*. In another photograph, Walkamoab balances on his peg leg, since the real one was amputated with an axe. In another picture, your grandfather stands lanky and tall beside a canoe in the Boundary Waters.

Before he'd decided how to devote his life, your grandfather sent your grandmother love-letters on postcards of peeled birchbark. According to family lore, his grandfather (whose parents sold him to a farm, given their poverty; your surname came from his owner) carved unbreakable chain-links from a single piece of wood.

As you sit with the photographs, you ask your grandfather whether he has written his stories: of his family and work (*humanitarian*, you soon learn the word) around the world. He says that actions speak louder than words, and he doesn't want to spend time *writing* when he might be *doing*. Housing foster children and gifting coats to huddles on street corners, he rarely has money, a pastor who is the son of a pastor.

You announce then, that you want to be like him, like your forebears: to be a pastor. You wait for him to clasp you in a grizzly hug, to say that's what he's always wanted. Instead, he answers with a question: Have you been *called*?

He says the word, which makes you think of telemarketers who interrupt at dinnertime, evoking your mother's wrath. You don't say this to your grandfather, because you sense gravity in his voice – a voice that has said his favorite ways to worship are silent prayer or a great big belly laugh. Working his way through college, he left school because he wasn't being taught what he thought he needed to learn: to understand the best of life, he needed to value what was considered otherwise. Without a lab coat or notebooks, he joined men living on streets, entered prisons and psychiatric wards in the guise of an inmate or patient, learning to listen.

You don't understand what your grandfather means by *called*, except that you have not been – and that everything seemed clear until he answered you with a question.

You continue thinking about this question after he asks,

What about your music?, when you accompany him and your sisters to an arts guild, deeper in the mountains, and watch him prepare microscope slides of citric acid for his class. He calls the workshop "Awe and Wonder." Toward midnight, after student artists view his slides, you follow him into a field, telescopes in tow. The lenses aren't needed for the Perseid Shower. You lie in grass and watch meteors stream across the sky, flailing tails of light, which resemble the microscope slides. The parallel patterns defy your teenaged reason.

You think about being *called*, after your grandfather has died, when all you want is an answer of what to do with your life, because music has betrayed you. Your voice is breaking, slowly, from a decade of over-singing in too many rehearsals, afternoons and evenings and weekends, with a girl's chorus in symphonies and orchestras, touring different States, through Europe and Asia. For children's roles in operas, you dress in petticoats and run across stage, past a painted park with governesses, singing numbers in Russian, or Italian vowels, trudging in a tattered cloak outside the court of a Pekinese princess, or guttural German, miked from offstage, near a ballet studio where you complete homework. At singing camp, operas are your bedtime stories, curled in your sleeping bag, waiting to hear what happens to Susanna or Lucia or the Queen of the Night. You memorize piece after piece, dynamics and lyrics and pronunciations, hone intonation and blend, and practice for Repertory Checks (the night before which you cram with your assigned quartet, seasonally, memorizing intricacies of each bar of each piece, retiring to bed past midnight with sheet music under your pillow). And although you're a Section Leader, a soloist and make a handful of friends, you're "the little giraffe" and get promoted too soon. The director pushes too hard, digs her nails into your cheeks to widen your smile (with metal braces), and screams if your vowels don't match the others, or if a chorister rubs eyes or scratches an ear; you're all required to stand with your hands at your side (*even if your parents stand up and take off their clothes, stark naked, in the middle of the audience, your eyes must never stray from the conductor!*). At camp and on tours, some of the older girls tease that you don't wear this or that fashion, that you don't shave your skin *there* or *here* (why are they looking? why do they care?), and when you get bronchitis and cough in the midst of Symphony Hall, a chorister kicks you in the back so hard your spine shudders, and you can't stop coughing, so you finally walk off stage and collapse in a sweat, with a temperature of 105.

After almost a decade, losing an octave of your range and being warned by an Ear, Nose, and Throat doctor that you may lose more, you decide to divorce music (at least, your voice) and tell your parents you want nothing to do with it ever, ever again.

But you can't do that. It's like trying to divorce a sense, like smell or taste or touch. And although your father isn't musical, he schedules your audition at the Conservatory, which you don't know about until he drives you there and begs, *Please don't give up your music.* He doesn't say the word, but you know it's like being *called*; your family believes in developing *God-given gifts.* You're not sure about gifts, or God, but despite your worn out voice, you are accepted, and since your teacher believes that singing is about love of music, he convinces you it will be worthwhile to learn to sing all over again (not so much the *what* of singing, but *how* and *why*), to go through the tedium of rebuild-

ing your range, which is like learning a new language. Like learning to speak after having been mute, only you are no longer a
child, and there is risk involved. Because your instrument isn't
perfectly healthy, and if you don't take care, you might do per-
manent damage.

You continue playing piano, in the midst of vocalizing and
practicing scales, studying scores, reviewing music theory and
history, pronouncing French, German, Italian, and other languages of your repertoire. Regardless, part of your heart is broken, as if music were a lover. You start searching for something
else and study subjects, like Spanish, which includes the verb *tocar*, meaning more than one thing: to play a musical instrument,
and to touch. You start following a different path, entirely away
from music.

Or so you think. Music plays between all lines of your
life, whether acknowledged or not. Traveling abroad, you hear
stories in Spanish more dangerous than weapons. Years pass.
Slowly, you come back to music like a prodigal daughter and pur-
sue piano, accompany and teach around the clock, overworking
a different part of your body: your hands. You ignore problems
because you don't have time, play and play, push and push, and
disregard symptoms as a matter of weakness, so soon your body
forgets how to be a body, and you can no longer play or do much
of anything: button your shirt, tie shoes, hold silverware. *She's
so young*, the doctors say, *her back is rebuilding and we can't
figure out why.* Your parents and sisters look at you befuddled-
ly and say, *You're not crooked*, until they admit: *You are.* After
months in decline, undergoing medical tests, getting misdiag-
nosed, shuttled between physical therapists and neurologists,

trying this and that approach, getting quieter and quieter as your body grows less and less mobile...

(*Lentamente*) ....*Lei m'intende? Mi chiamano.... Vivo sola, soletta, lá in una bianca cameretta; guardo sui tetti e in cielo. Ma quando vien lo sgelo il primo sole è mio.... (senza regore di tempo con naturalezza:) Altro di me no le saprei narrare. Sono la sua vicina che la vien fuori d'ora a importunare...*

With lost tactile sense, you walk blindfolded, with taped and reshaped hands, learn Braille, search with your fingers for pairable shapes in boxes of children's toys, trying to connect something essential that has become disjoined.

Although silent, your voice doesn't betray you this time.

You rely on it to lead you home – even if not singing, but speaking into a voice-activated computer. It's a bit like modulation: if the song changes keys around the whole Circle of Fifths, it will lead you back (away from and returning) home. To the home key.

The key for the lock –

Articulations and re-articulations force you to consider the double nature of literature and language, less its written medium than its oral origins. And although yours is a different *call* than your grandfather's, and your faith no longer fits anything singular (because you trust questions more than answers now, though maybe he'd say that's exactly the point), you're gleaning some sense of what he meant. Progress to you is unlearning as much as learning, unknotting what has been tied, so your story unravels (the meaning of *dénouement*, after all). In fits and starts, you listen in a new way to words, against silence, as if that were your call – where wonder is elusive and temporal as music.

This sound comes to the surface, then sinks, then rises to the surface and floats, then dissolves. To hear and live it, moment by moment – you give thanks that it's possible to wander, wondering, at all.

Ut queant laxis

*L*ook! (at captions in galleries, she glimpses): the sun is halved in one painting and elsewhere shines whole, above the horizon line. Placards refer back and forth, where curators have planned a course through display after display, on podiums behind glass lit indirectly: YOU ARE HERE. In the Seljuk Period. She finds herself (breathing) at a fork in the road, beside chess pieces (complete save for a single pawn, "check-mate" from *sha-mat*, "I give up," *Iran XII century AD*), queens & rooks, square by square, once maneuvered for kingdoms and princesses, beside an elderly couple who hovers over the explanation, whispering, *So that's where and when it began* (as if beginnings are singular; as if knowing makes a difference; as if chansons shaped like hearts mean more than unrecorded words):

Where did it begin, & with whom?

Round and round, she goes among Rustam & Isfandiyar & Simurgh & Firdausi & Demotte & pedar & madar & baradar (Faar & Mor & Eva & Una & Avra & You) who seep from fired tiles & calligraphed niches & woven carpets, all tangled together like vines in a jungle – she tries to

read the webs of script, to unravel their stories. She's looking for an inroad, to follow any beginning that can be traced
from here & back again, re-raveled with other beginnings as
endings, not hidden but revealed to suggest what came before
with after. *I need to hear this music inside*, she thinks, *What re-
sides in bodies, like houses shelter* (rooms, "stanzas," constitut-
ing homes on ever-covered foundations)? *How did all come
to be, worlds, every day dawning, sinking into dusk and rising
again, granted and taken for blessed, or cursed?*

In the middle of the gallery, she pauses (among those
who come to go, enticed by Michelangelo) & thinks: *Where
am I*, who everything fills with wonder, which often brings
euphoria, but sometimes makes her sad. She cares too much,
she's been told, for love of living, for love of loving; for love
of visiting shimmering miniaturist paintings from the epic
Shahnama, so fine and detailed, painted with brushes made
from hair on the bellies of squirrels and kittens, & calligraphy
sweeping like Shivac arms in a penumbra of fiery dance; for
love of circumambulating galleries like gated chambers of a
temple, & of navigating hope by love – the possibility of beginning anew:

Homing: Honing: Home:

Solve polluti

Home. They were moving. Homing. It was hard to know where, exactly, because they were on a journey. West from the Midwest, Eva and Una followed Mor and Faar, and went where they were told. They left behind fields that glimmered like oceans in summer, where in winter Faar's barn hid under snow so its roof sailed like an upside-down skiff at sea.

It was summer now. Beyond cornfields, sandy hills came first in the distance. Rivers roamed. Cranes congregated in lavender-green marshes. The birds danced on spindly legs and flew toward clouds. Watching them disappear, the four-year-olds smelled displaced brine, feeling the pull of tides without knowing the War-to-End-All-Wars was spreading across oceans.

Onward, in fields of sage-stock, the girls found grains ground with ghost-blue shells. One shell was whole and didn't belong. Without a whatnot shelf in their migrating home, the sisters carried it: cradled it in joined palms, held it between their ears, listened with reverence to its sighs. The sounds washed delicately, like a dove's elusive coo. They tried with patience to understand and become susceptible to the quiet call. Summoning sounds, they continued west toward sunset, holding the coiled calcium to

their ears, waiting for they knew not what. Una and Eva combined
what they heard; their lives grew ever more composite.

Above a dry inland sea, pelicans, storks, and gulls flew. The
sisters listened to their shell and felt a need to dig. They had no
stick to direct their course, but their fingers sifted to caress grainy
clusters. Deeper, deeper. Unearthing pebbles and scum, they
found a bone. It was from the pelvis of some forgotten creature,
bleached and worn. The girls didn't dig deeper to find the rest of
a body. Their satisfaction was singular. A bone wasn't yet specified
as attached to another. Eva and Una put it with their shell, not for
that to summon sound, but rather because both objects had been
lost like Holde and might hold her hidden heart.

Traveling under clouds like sails, the family bypassed plains
and peaks, navigating west and north. The last leg of their journey brought them to a valley. The family settled in an abandoned
farmhouse, in an abandoned orchard. In those first difficult days,
the girls yearned for sleep so bread and molasses might come to
them in dreams, without ration. Deprivation carved their senses,
as Faar and Mor foraged for food and water. Mor collected root-
stalks and berries. On a charred hearth, Faar browned fish on
flames. Eva and Una picked meat off thinly branched bones, between sips of spruce tea.

The sisters missed home. They wanted to return. Between
star-hushed nights, something or someone kept them safe enough
to stay. One-thousand-and-one feet above the sea, rattlers hid under blackberry brambles and could have bitten, but bushes provided only beads of sweet juice. Poison oak scrambled up rocks and

trees and also could have afflicted. But the red-and-green ternate leaves entwined lilies with congeniality, without threat.

Slowly, Faar patched the decrepit farmstead, the *bøndegard*, as autumn descended and brought a wild harvest. The sisters splashed in leaves, crimson and gold, among fallen fruits. They looked for pairs, like they appeared: twin wild plums, twin acorns, twin berries, twin nuts, twin almonds. There was an old wive's tale about twin fruits, twin children, and second sight, which the girls had not yet learned; nor did they know that in another time and place, twin girls and their mothers were killed because it was believed that a man could not plant more than one seed. In this time and place, the girls ate heartily in ignorance, unappreciative of their luxurious survival.

A fruit that they had not seen before—in the shape of a bloated heart, plump like an apple but pumpkin-orange—grew on one of the trees outside the window. Faar had no word for it and adopted the classification that a neighbor offered: *per-sim-mon*. The girls learned its name and rolled the syllables over their tongues. Its skin was leathery and tough, its leaves stiff and brittle.

They learned to wait for the orbs to ripen, placing them in basins with apples and pears until each softened and lost its pucker. Skinning and slicing the fresh flesh, they put it on their tongues to slither down their throats. Mor boiled the surplus and stirred its bubbling pulp into jam; with eggs, milk, walnuts, and raisins into persimmon pudding; into biscuits that steamed when the sisters broke open hot crusts at the same moment.

There were also pies combining persimmons with fruits

from the orchards. The farm grew *epler, päerer, aprikøs,* and *vøl-nøtter* on gnarled trees. Some trunks had holes for hiding found objects: the shell and bone from the in-land seas, yarn and needles, and wrappers from candy, which the family could afford only at Christmas.

When Faar pruned trees, branch stubs seemed like fists shaking at parched clouds. Roots lay shallow from drought and sucked sustenance only from the surface. Mor made the twins dig for water together, as if they might find twice as much. "The devil works through idle hands," she repeated in their shared tongue, when the *datters* didn't keep their fingers busy. Her industrious digits knitted sweaters, socks, scarves, mittens, and *hardanger.* In I-o-w-a, Mor had raised her own sheep and woven wool with shuttles, marrying wefts and warps. Her loom was left behind when the family moved West, but every item made by Mor was meant to last.

While Mor mended, the girls helped Faar sow fields. Days were work, but nights the *datters* wandered with him away from the house, to look for stars. Faar knew legends of the constellations from his *faar* before him, looked for Auriga through a telescope ordered from Sears & Roebuck, and told the story of the goat who carried twins and looked for shipwrecked sailors. He also had ordered a seed scope, to see the grains of his crops and to show his girls miniature worlds. It didn't matter what was magnified, he said, as long as his *datters* knew that everything could be perceived up close, not only *en vei,* from multiple points of view.

Eva and Una received their own scope, called *ka-lei-do,*

which was pebbled with color and twistable: stars of green, rinsed red and gold. Splintering shapes mixed together, overlapped, made new hues and forms, and transformed the world the viewers knew. Their eyes needed time to adjust and absorb each reconfiguration, which was new only because the sisters hadn't known it before and so did not take it for granted.

New sights were like that. They introduced contrasts and definitions. They distinguished wonders: awe from horror, grief from joy.

Resonare fibris

With each passing year, Eva pruned boughs so they wouldn't break, watched them thicken and filter sunlight through laced leaves. At harvest, apples dripped like rain, piling the ground faster than they could be picked: raw and for preserves, apple butter, cider, vinegar, applejack, brandy. Hauling them back to the A-frame, she used an old press, pots and pans of sizable shapes to distill, ferment, and make all manner of products, to barter alongside notions and knickknacks for clothes and food at a roadside stand – collecting nothing to keep, but to restore or re-make, then give away.

Deep in the roots of her family tree, some daughters (sisters, later mothers and grandmothers) had received seeds inside swatches of calico from a traveler who had followed branches of the Old Northwest by boat and barefoot, toting rotten windfalls and coffee sacks of seeds, in two lashed canoes, wearing a tin dipper for a hat, nursing old orchards, pushing West to plant new ones. During nights when the traveler came to Eva in dreams, she learned to drink snow, to subsist off wild nuts and berries, to find salves in herbs, to stay warm without a fire because mosquitoes and other insects were fatefully drawn to flames.

After months, after years sped their course, or slowed (whatever distilled his molasses voice, beard of nested birds, skin so weathered it couldn't be pierced by a serpent): Eva started seeing him during the day. He helped her to tend the orchard, and after it grew, she waited long enough in willowy grasses with the sun warming her cheeks, until he'd amble through marigolds or paddle around the bend of the river in his double-canoe, ready to retrieve her offered bushels and pecks. Never staying longer than the exchange required, he made exceptions only to check trees for blight, mind her pruning and grafting, and unload new seeds.

His visits were never predictable but for one thing: he never neglected to bring a chapter of his favorite book, disordered, because he'd lent other sections to those he met before her. And hope of learning what happened next in the shuffled story, more than the propensity to plant, kept Eva's orchard thriving.

And when he stopped coming, and she only heard his molasses voice by memory or mistakenly, when birds warbled, she started making trips out of the valley to scatter seeds in fruitless spots, thinking that maybe by going through his motions, she'd glean the end of the story about the man who'd never been found, whose grave held no bones, who was sighted two decades after his death on Lookout Mountain: "a phantom sprung from the moon."

Avra remembered the phrase for the moon-sprung man more than her own grandfather, whom she'd never met and knew nothing about, but a legend and his initials, *M.E.* Her mother, a legend too, until recently. Something grafted all these lives, from letters (now lost) and torn stories (between lines, in margins), until slowly Avra realized how her story, how his story (any story – how yours, how mine) can grow palpable enough to be handled and mishandled, as the storyteller herself retreats somewhere in the map.

Blossoms burst from her lips. Withering limbs silhouetted winter light. Ghosting into fog, sun crept through a veil of gray, rippling down wrinkled cliffs. Birds trembled. Avra smelled pine and fire in place of her ears and eyes. A flurry. No longer numb, but tingling, she inhaled earth, bark, wood mixed with the sweet rot of apples, and again wondered if the smell came from inside her, if she wasn't transparent and could generate a scent, refract light, disturb a breeze. How was her spirit shaped? She followed the fog until a figure emerged.

Resonare fibris – Labii reatum

She followed the fog until a figure emerged. In Golden Gate Park, he appeared out of nowhere: tattered, with long white hair hanging down his chest like a beard, pushing a shopping cart. He offered an apple, without a word. Avra could barely murmur a sound before he disappeared, and fog engulfed her view.

She started to shake more than shiver. Almost wanting to follow him, she walked briskly in the other direction, glancing over her shoulder. He'd seemed real – there had been a shopping cart, for God's sake – where did *that* go? Her mind thudded, remembering her mother one night, two months before, when Avra had sat huddled in a corner, shaking, stuttering, *Don't know if.* Isabel had embraced her and said, *Yes, you can. You're still here.*

Here. Here. "You're still here," Avra whispered. Her warm breath puffed visibly in front of her face. The mist made her aware of moistness on her cheeks, her socks' dampness, the chill. She looked over her shoulder, then down at her empty mangled hand.

It was still there – her hand – newly reconstructed with two toes, grafted where her fingers should've been. And she was still coming to grips with the fire that had crushed her fingers, caused her husband's death and their home's collapse, leaving her to raise their four-year-old daughter, under the roof of a woman she barely knew: her mother. Isabel. Twenty years had passed since her mother had "died." Instead of dying, however, Isabel had undergone a series of conversions, lived in a convent and a few ashrams, while Avra's father had concealed her secret, maintaining intermittent contact, until a heart attack caused his real death. His lawyer continued to update Isabel and notified her about Avra's freakish fire. Then, Avra received a phone call from a woman who said: "I'm ready in my journey of faith to be a mother and grandmother. Give me a chance; who else do you have?" Needing to physically recover, pay debts and raise a young child, Avra hadn't seen an option other than moving in with her divinely-demented mother.

A horn honked. Headlights beamed through fog, even at midafternoon. Avra didn't know where to go. Having finished her shift at the museum, as a part-time gallery guard, she was headed home – not home: Isabel's house. "The house should follow a natural course to decay," Isabel had explained her philosophy of maintenance (essentially: disrepair), "not from neglect, but with attention to basic precepts of traditional Japanese architecture, and the process of returning a structure to its original elements."

The stoplight changed. Avra crossed the street, thinking more about her mother's domestic philosophy. An unlicensed consultant had advised Isabel to rebuild the structure with a thatched roof and bamboo walls, lighter than stucco, more economical, easily assembled and disassembled, and flexible in earthquakes. That reconstruction hadn't yet happened. Avra could only await the house's collapse.

On the next block, shop windows framed displays: videos in front of Chaplin's hat-and-mustache and a Kurosawa dreamscape; a linen table for two; train-tracks traversing slopes around a miniature town. Avra loitered. With Carrie at the Rahads, she felt less inclined to go directly to Isabel's house. Instead, she wanted to go inside somewhere – anywhere – to get out of the chill, to feel some surge of warmth.

On the next block, a wooden sign hung over a door: *Books Within Books*. The window hosted an arrangement like a house of cards. Shouldering the door, Avra opened it. A bell clinked.

Disheveled shelves overflowed with stacked spines. White flags with subject headings jutted from sections. The room smelled musty with damp warmth. On the uneven hardwood floor, aged fruit crates with faded black lettering bulged with more books. A young man with tousled hair and goatee looked up from behind the counter.

"Today's your lucky day," he said in a nasal voice.

She smiled and peered at the shelves, skimming titles.

He glanced down at her hand, a moment too long to go unnoticed.

"You haven't visited before," he stated as if he remembered everyone who came to the shop. "Let me recommend something."

He stepped from behind the counter and approached her. His dark green suit looked faded, two sizes too big. "I'm proud of my stock, if you like used books – *books within books*, you know?" He pulled a text from the shelf, flipped it open, and pointed to underlined sentences and marginal scribbles. "This is what I like. Twice the story: writer's and reader's." He shut the book and shelved it. She caught him looking at her hand again. "That must be hard," he said, opening and closing his left fingers.

She gaped at his forthrightness.

"My uncle lost his in Vietnam. The thing is, after that, he didn't let go, as if all his demons were right in his hand, holding him in some grip."

She looked away, wary of his confidence and presumptions. She wanted to browse books in peace.

"He should've just let go. My uncle, that is." He shook his intact hands, then pushed forward both palms, like a mime. "I know that's easy for me to say." He dropped his hands to his sides. "Remember what I said," he said. "About this being your lucky day?"

She nodded, uneasily.

He scanned another shelf, then slipped out a tome. "You haven't read this, have you?"

She glanced at the spine: *The Street Enters the House.* "No."

He pulled off the dustjacket, where a reproduced illuminated hand with syllables on the palm and digits replaced the author's photo. Avra looked at the base of the ring finger and read: *E, la, mi.* "I think the author uses a pseudonym," said the

bookseller. "I heard an interview on public radio a while back."
He flipped through pages, enough for her to notice typographic
acrobatics, constellated images, arabesquing lists, letters and
numbers. He stopped on a more linear page and said, "Read
that aloud."

"Aloud?" Avra glanced to see if anyone was in the shop.
They were alone. The text under his finger read, "She sighed," on
a page with lines so short, white space dominated. She thought
of a snow drift, blanketing the remaining letters.

"Just read this part," he said. "It's not like anybody's listening." He glanced down at her hands. "I'll hold it for you. See
where it takes you."

"Where it takes me?"

He nodded.

Avra inhaled deeply, regretting her predicament, wishing she'd bypassed the bookstore. To get it over with, she started to read: Arturo didn't know how to respond. He wanted to say
words but didn't know if she wanted to hear. Avra stopped.

"Keep going," coaxed the bookseller. "You're doing great."

—I guess you weren't...wouldn't be...aren't....

—Not that, now.

—May I ask...

—What?

—When?

—This...may not, she looked away. —end. It may worsen. I
mean, everything depends.

—On?

—The outside getting in.

—Into what? Do you...?

—...I? she laughed. He thought her eyes looked sad. *—That question is for anyone. Do you?*

—What? I don't understand. What riddle is....?

She looked up to the trees, to the light. He hesitated, wanting to answer her questions.

—You seem well, he said and his gaze moved down her face, and lower. Her eyes shot to meet his.

—I have to go, she said.

Avra looked up. The line was timely. "*I* have to go," she repeated.

"A bit more," said the bookseller.

She sighed but read, swiveled and started to squirm away. Pigeons dispersed to the sky. As he longingly watched her dodge toward ashes and oaks, he noticed her tilt. She scuttled, not quite vertically. She shrank at a slant toward the brush, and his squint veered from her toward marble heroes, plaques, crumbs, rooks, castles, pawns & again, her sliver – and he felt recur a feeling from a visit to Pisa, that tipped his answers toward questions, of whether he himself was straight or crooked.

"Enough." The bookseller shut the book. "So." His eyes squinted. "You have ten seconds to decide."

"To decide what?"

"The magic word."

"What?"

"'What' IS the magic word! Well done."

"Pardon?"

"The book is yours."

"I don't want to buy it."

"You don't have to. It's yours." He shoved it into her right hand. Her body-weight shifted like a scale, teetering to one side. "Once a month, I pick a lucky customer to give them a book. You never know whether you're the one, until you're it."

She was silent, thinking, *How the hell will I carry this home, let alone read it?* She hadn't read a whole book since the fire.

He shrugged his shoulders, "Happy American Heart Month."

"What? I can't take it."

"No, it's *yours* now, whether or not you want it." He laughed, but her face didn't change. "No strings attached. It's yours. Just tell people to patronize the store, and they can be my next lucky customers."

The book almost fell out of her right hand. She shifted, so it caught on her hip. He kept speaking, absorbed in his own words, as she sidled up to the counter and hefted the book slowly onto the ledge. "Really, I can't take it," she interrupted.

His face wrinkled in agitation. "Please don't leave it here. Wait a sec –"

She forced a smile but turned away, getting angry, not knowing what held her here. She looked toward the windows, grey, like smoke. The apartment. The fire. Her mind raced to the day when she'd returned from work to find flames billowing from their apartment window. Stephen had died of smoke inhalation. He'd stopped breathing. She'd lost part of her hand, crushed by a falling beam when she ran inside. A firefighter rescued her. Carrie had been at daycare. The cause of the blaze hadn't been found, but the local paper reported that the negligent landlord owned a number of properties that were "disasters waiting to happen."

"Here." The bookseller stepped in front of her and handed her a bookmark that matched the cover. "Please take *The Street Enters the House*."

She looked from him, to the bookmark and book, waiting on the counter. Awkwardly, she uncinched her Velcro waistpack, which expanded to twice its size. Although the book heaved, it fit perfectly. All she needed to do was leave the store and give it to a passerby or drop it on the curb. "Thanks," she said, flatly. "I'll recommend your bookstore."

"Do that! Please do that. And come back when you've finished *The Street Enters the House*."

Yes, she nodded, thinking *no*.

A bell clinked as she left the store.

She lumbered up the block but didn't drop the book, still thinking of the fire. At the next intersection, the slope rose to highrises like luminaries. Without knowing why, she followed the lights – in the opposite direction of Isabel's house. By the time she reached the first highrise, her limbs ached. She stopped by a glass kiosk flanked with flowers.

"Hello," said the florist. "Can I help you find something?"

Avra glanced at a bucket of irises, recalling that Stephen

had brought her a bouquet at Carrie's birth. She'd never brought him flowers in the hospital – he hadn't made it there in time.

"Miss?" The florist pointed. "Do you want some?"

"What?" Avra looked around at fog.

"Irises, or maybe mums?"

"Yes."

"Both?"

Avra remembered her wallet, holding $1.34.

"They're a dollar per stem."

"One iris."

Avra removed change from her Velcroed pouch and sorted it awkwardly on the counter. A revolving rack held palm-sized envelopes and tags: *Happy Birthday, Get Well Soon, For Your Anniversary.*

"A card?"

"No," Avra's stomach knotted. Who would she write a card to? Besides, writing her name (if only signing debit card receipts) was humiliating. Before the injury, cashiers had never checked her signature, but now nobody believed that she was herself until she held up her reconstructed hand. Then they believed it, but Avra didn't.

The woman handed over pennies with the plastic-wrapped bouquet.

Avra stepped back, not knowing where to go. People flowed past as if she were a stone in a river. The fog's chill made her shiver. The heft of the book weighed down her hip. She suddenly needed a bathroom.

So she walked. To a crosswalk, to a building, following halls. She found herself in an elevator, then another hallway, looking left to right, forgetting the bathroom. Beeping monitors pulsed. Televisions hummed. Doors framed glimpses of tangled tubes, intravenous lines, oxygen drips and ventilators. Her breath grew long and heavy; her heart felt parched and throbbed for air. She leaned against a wall to keep from falling.

"Can I help you?"

Avra raised her head. A young male nurse faced her.

"I...I'm –" Avra didn't know what to say.

"Do you want to leave flowers for someone?" he prompted.

"Yes."

"The patient's name?" he asked, smiling.

Avra looked down the hall, not saying a word.

His brow furrowed.

"I didn't – don't know why I'm here." She thrust her flower into his hands. "If anyone needs this," she didn't finish her sentence, just turned and started hurriedly walking away.

Not the right person, not the right time.

She retraced her steps down the corridor. At the elevators, she pushed the down-pointing arrow, repeatedly. A panel of floor numbers illuminated distant locations of other elevators. The air seemed too warm. Nauseating. She saw an exit sign and took the stairs down ten flights. Given the ballast-like weight of the book, her lope was crooked the whole way down.

She lumbered out of the hospital, engulfed by darkness.

Like other days she'd spent in San Francisco, night had fallen behind a veil of fog, warping her sense of time. A line of cars crept through the Slow Zone, laced in mist. Headlights blurred a blinking electric red hand. She didn't know what time it was. A public bus steered to the curb and opened its doors. As soon as the light changed, she dashed across the crosswalk and boarded the bus.

She couldn't sit without removing the bulging book. The bus puttered down the hill before it went up again, stopping every few corners, as her new weight bounced on her lap. *The Street Enters the House.* She examined the cover, drenched with colors portraying what-seemed-to-be a woman in blue painted from behind, standing at a warped balcony, facing a city square with a riot of red horses and bodies, surrounded by incongruously slanted, brightly-colored houses.

Avra used her right hand to flip forward a few pages. The bookmark slipped to her lap. Like the dust jacket, it pictured an illuminated hand marked with syllables: *C, fa, ut...* Intrigued, she opened the book to the middle, tilting it awkwardly against the seat in front of her, and started to read: "Arturo Francamano heard the rickity crackity thrum that churned motions of a notion, rain against some grain, and a taste: *wet wheat*, as he gazed at fields outside glass."

Labii reatum – Resonare fibris – Mira gestorum

Arturo Francamano heard the rickity crackity thrum that churned motions of a notion, rain against some grain, and a taste: *wet wheat*, as he gazed at fields outside glass. He was riding a train. Thirstily imbibing sights and sounds, he imagined himself atop the passenger car drenched by whirs, clackings, puffs; as gusts saturated his skin and suit, he shook sopped hair and cupped his hands. Rain streaked his cheeks, unquenched as tears. Batting his lashes he spied gray plumes and metal bars that hooked over the roof into a ladder, for his descent. Down, down, down. He clenched each rung; meadows blurred from the speed and from falling drops. Arturo held fast to the crossbars. Slowly, he stretched his hand toward waving wheat. Once, not far enough. A second stretch. Chaff slipped between his fingers. Then. A stalk whipped in the wind as he clung to it and to the train. He drew it to his mouth, laid the wet wheat on his tongue, and chewed. Rickity crackity. Thrum slid down his throat, as sounds and sights hazed his senses and sorted grains into a *meal to feel*: texture, not mere subsistence, as he imagined a new carminative concoction of *noodles, seared anise stars and sesame, slurped while shaking a rattle to play a patter of rain* – an addition to the ever-evolving menu for his restaurant, The Holy Palate.

Arturo reached again to grab wet wheat, but his hand hit plastic and polyester. A chair, a row in a car of a train. Blue, gray, and orange plaid fabric. He rubbed his eyes. His face, hair, and hands were dry in a seat beside a woman (who was reading) and a window (shielding them both from the storm). He glanced at the woman, then back toward fields rippling, bending, curling under sleet and, ahead, to a smokestack purring steam. In the fog, threads of roads danced.

The train curved and approached a railroad crossing, where semaphore lights blinked yellow and red. Striped slats barred a blue stationwagon, whose wiping windshield appeared to blush. Arturo considered the aura and audibility of the train as the procession approached and passed, changing sound in departing. Gold, red, green. Leaves then lightning flashed autumn winter spring summer – back to fall's harvestable *wet wheat*, which Arturo needed to rename in lexicon of his own making, if he hoped to offer it to customers without context, disguised, to nip their presumptions into buds.

More rain blurred the outside view; water droplets beaded into rivulets; and obscurity focused Arturo to the point of distraction, by a fly buzzing, buzzing, splatting. Above the inside ledge of the window, it stuck like a bitty-black star to which he raised his fingers, but stopped. He considered the possibility of living inside-out; however, since the fly evidently was not living at all, Arturo focused on *whywherewhat* its paralyzed fate might lend him. Having watched the collision at that point of co-ordination where invisible lines from sides intersected, he retraced the path of the flown fly to a grid only he could see, through closed eyes. Arturo clenched his lids tightly, so stars began to pop and shine. And through closed eyes, he watched the black beady bug enlarge, inflate to pterodactylic proportions as invertebrate features grew voluptuous and vein-laced, crusted, compounded; wings hinged to exoskeletal thorax and abdomen with iridescent humps, six jointed-stalk legs, and two tentacle-like antennae *on a bed of steamed spinach or seaweed*, he thought, *something slimy to complement the crunch; green to underscore the black and iridescence; and heated to contrast coolness. How might I fake the fly, as a feast?*, he pondered the transformation, since his restaurant did not serve things as themselves, but as representations.

To undermine diners' expectations, meals were titled by unrecognizable names, and ingredients blended to bake unassumed shapes, sizes, temperatures, and textures – anything to maximize the *feeling* of a dish. The provocation of feelings was Arturo's calling, after all; he was sensitive to textures since they'd been his prime criterion in judging food. Since birth, he had anosmia and rarely smelled or tasted (the senses were physiologically related; his first recognition came at twenty-three); but slowly, his proclivities had led him to cook meals-to-feel, even as he continued working at a laboratory breeding thousands of *Drosophila melanogaster*. The most versatile and maneuverable of all flying machines – hovering, accelerating, decelerating, rolling, looping and landing, *Fruit flies*. They defied laws of quasi steady-state aerodynamics and encouraged him to depart from conventions. He painted their wings with a platinum porphyrin dissolved in an oxygen-permeable polymer (a phosphorescent compound) to illuminate their delicate mesh

movements with ultraviolet light, in a way that even ten years after he first bred them, made him tingle as he thought of pressures
over entire surfaces of things and the search to understand those
stresses, as he looked at the splatted fly on the window of a train and
considered the forces that killed it.

Speeding on its course, the train continued to prod Arturo
to move, to raise his fingers and touch the thrum where the bug
no longer buzzed. He wanted to hold it closer toward his eyes then
place it under magnification by a microscope, at his home beside
glass slides, boxes, labels, pins, and books. He considered whether
it was arbitrary enough to suggest to Nova, his lover and confidant,
who tape-recorded (because of her injured hands, which hindered
her sense of touch) tales – one-act plays – dependent on his daily choice of three subjects. He didn't need to bring home physical
evidences, only names of nouns as plain as *soup, soldiers, & stones*,
which Nova would knit with verbs to reveal hidden connections.

(A sidebar of marginalia directed Avra to turn to another
page, where she found one such play:

STONE SOUP;
OR, A RECIPE PLIED WITH PLIGHT

(A TRAGICOMEDY IN ONE ACT)

The page included stage directions and a cast of characters: NARRATOR, FIRST SOLDIER, SECOND SOLDIER, THIRD SOLDIER, OLD
MAN, OLD WOMAN, WELL-WOMAN, MIRANDA, BELLY-DANCER... Avra

stopped reading, deciding to return to the play later, flipping back to:) *Would she want to write of the fly?* In the midst of the storm, he considered the idea and touched the insect. It fell off the glass and left scum. Arturo followed the drop, lowered, and tottered his head under the row. He rummaged among candy wrappers, paper case of a straw, stiff-wadded tissue, crumbs, and a stainless spoon (whose scoop turned him so he considered momentarily *upside down life?*), but his mind continued to host the image of the fly, stronger than his own concave face.

(Avra glanced out the window, as the bus steered its course, still some distance from Isabel's house. Dreading arrival, Avra kept reading for distraction:) The bug fit among his edible arthropods. The Menu for his restaurant was inspired by all conceivable subjects, animate and inanimate, art architecture music transportation technology historical physical chemical biological ecological astronomical noumenalogical and phenomenological sciences not yet named. Like the grandiose gene pool whose winding stairways of As Ts Cs and Gs had influenced his ideas, the Menu was encoded in language whose alphabet combined, recombined, mutated, bred and was growing fast past his last count, of some thirty-three hundred pages. Arturo and Nova had brainstormed that much. In addition to writing one-act plays, Nova was his "intrapreneurial" partner (they had patented the term "business-within-a-business") and together, the couple had conceived and hybridized new meals. Each day, as knowledge was discovered, evolved, and expanded, they felt surer that their grand scheme might succeed *wherehowwhen* experiments stretched far enough from the restaurant, through apprenticed chefs, through the multi-volume cookbook and ever-expanding dictionary of textures. Then, the effort that had begun in a private kitchen, partly from Arturo's anosmia and partly to accommodate Nova's intangible abilities, might change the world.

As the images and words whirled in his mind like buzzing bugs, the train curved, and the moving window momentarily hosted two views: Arturo and the woman reading beside him, plus slivered sun. The light splayed more beams through the storm and illuminated another meal, his favorite fig butter with salsa, poached eggs and rye, which Arturo had eaten ten years before on a park bench, beside three old men playing chess near a path, where he glimpsed the young woman who he'd met the year before that.

Arturo dropped his sandwich. He sprinted toward the path on which she walked. Nova stopped and turned to walk in the direction from which she'd come. But he'd already reached her side.

—*Remember?* he asked.

She moved her hands behind her back, glanced at him and stones in the road, and said, —*Phosphorescent drosophilae and....*

—*Framed motions.*

She looked away. —*You talked about going backwards, to go forwards....*

—*I tried your number,* he gushed. *When someone finally answered, he said you were....*

—*Yes,* she nodded, looking back.

Both of them shifted nervously.

—*How is your animation?* he asked.

—*My anima-...oh? Not me, my project.* She glanced at the

men playing chess, a retriever curled among legs, pigeons feather-
ing statues, and verdigris urns that flanked the square. She sighed,
—*De Corporis Fabrica.*

Arturo had forgotten the meaning and didn't know how to respond. He wanted to ask but hesitated. —*What? I guess you weren't...
wouldn't be...aren't....*

—*Not that, now.*

—*May I ask...*

—*What?*

—*When?*

—*This...may not*, she looked away. —*end. It may worsen. I
mean, everything depends.*

—*On?*

—*The outside getting in.*

—*Into what? Do you...?*

—*...I?* she laughed. He thought her eyes looked sad.

—*That question is for anyone. Do you?*

—*What? I don't understand. What riddle is....?*

She looked up to the trees, to the light. He hesitated, wanting
to answer her questions.

—*You seem well*, he said and his gaze moved down her face,
and lower. Her eyes shot to meet his.

—*I have to go*, she said.

She swiveled and started to squirm away. Pigeons dispersed
to the sky. As he longingly watched her dodge toward ashes and
oaks, he noticed her tilt. She scuttled, not quite vertically. She shrank
at a slant toward the brush, and his squint veered from her toward

the trio of seniors, marble heroes, plaques, crumbs, rooks, castles, pawns & again, her sliver – and he felt recur a feeling from a visit to Pisa, that tipped his answers toward questions, of whether he himself was straight or crooked.

And as Arturo lost himself in his thoughts-relative-to-time-in-the-train, he scurried to the place between trees where Nova had disappeared, on muddy dirt. At his feet beside footprints, twigs, and leaves, he glimpsed a small box. He picked it up and rubbed off mud. It was palm-sized, square, wooden, and inlaid with dark and light woods in a geometric maze. He removed the lid. Another box hid inside, decorated in the same pattern with a similar lid, which he removed to find another box, another smaller box and others, encased and differing only by size. The last, tiniest boxlid was sealed.

A clock chimed, in Arturo's recollection. He looked toward the peals, twelve, from a clock on a gate around a carousel. The ring enclosed carved mares. *Open at Two* read the sign. Plop. Plop. His attention followed the sound, a third plop, the arced path of a stone, a hand that threw the rocks. A boy. The boy continued to throw stones. Plop, plop, plop. Arturo watched pebbles propelled to water, rippling in widening circles. The rings intersected. Observing closely, he raised the box toward his eyes and....*where, why, what... could it be?...*

Arturo smelled a scent.

He'd never known the sense but guessed its name, as he inhaled cedar. A new perception! And in the moment he realized his gain, he shoved the box in his pocket and started to run. To find Nova. He had to find Nova. Sunlight winked on the lake, another stone splashed, and Arturo pivoted toward the carousel, the clock, the trees, branches and leaves; past begonias bees strollers hop-scotchers jacks swings&slides toward leashes dogs "here" and "fetch" and the plinking tune of a trolley. He *ranranran* all the while leaping and looking, for someone he trusted only by sense. He panted, breathless, searching until he saw....

—*Sir*, the wind whispered, as leaves and light flitted. Arturo turned to find no one, pivoted again, slowly rotating under the trees, branches, overarching canopy. Filtered light, spinning. As he whirled, he closed his eyes, opened and closed them again, as sun streaked his cheeks with warmth, opening and closing; he batted his lashes as colors blurred, and he blinked blue, gray, and orange. Plaid. He gazed at the glowing grid wondrously as it tilted. His head rested; velour cradled his cheek. The train gently rocked him. Arturo's eyelids started sinking again. The softness moved.

—Sir, *please*. Arturo turned toward the whisper. He blinked at mauve.

—Sir, I'm sorry to disturb you, said a mouth coming into focus on the face of a woman holding a book. —Sir...sir? You seem to have fallen asleep on my shoulder.

Arturo gasped, lifted his head, and straightened against his seat. The plaid shifted from diamonds to squares. —Oh, he puffed. —What, who? How...sorry. It...it must be the rain.

She smiled and said, —Everyone needs rest, now and then. She opened her book and returned to reading (while the bus driver called "Ortega." Avra looked up. *Where am I?* She glanced down at her book, then at her bus stop, and tried to cram the text into her waist pack. *Wait, wait. Just a little more time.* The new book refused to fit. She tried to jam the seams, as the doors began to close. "Wait!" she called aloud. The driver didn't hear and steered the bus from the curb.

Backtracking to the house, on foot, her body felt crooked from the imbalanced weight. Isabel opened the door and just looked at her. "It's eight o'clock," she said. "Where on earth did you go?"

"I got on the wrong bus," Avra lied. *The Street Enters the House* heaved in her side-pouch, but she didn't want to remove it, lest Isabel pester her with questions.

They walked through the house to the kitchen, where Carrie was eating cereal. Avra didn't have energy to argue.

"Hi, Mom," Carrie grinned, chewing another spoonful.

Milk dribbled down her chin. Isabel brushed her own chin, and Carrie dabbed hers. Avra watched bewilderedly as her daughter and mother exchanged signs. Isabel's small, wrinkled fingers fluttered toward a teacup, bright against her aqua sarong. A headscarf fanned her curls. This attire – or the saris, kimonos, and wraps of kente (stamped with the *sankofa* bird, which Isabel had explained "looks backward") – didn't correspond with Avra's blurred memories from early childhood: her mother in housedresses or church clothes with white gloves, a quarter-century ago, when Avra had been told that her mother had died. There had even been a funeral. The finality had been Isabel's wish – "your father needed to tell you something that wouldn't make you feel like you were my reason for leaving,

since you weren't, nor was he." She had changed her name
from Alice to Isabel, not only to mean "consecrated to God,"
Avra guessed, but also to keep from being found.

"I burned marigolds this morning for Stephen," Isabel
said, referring to her dead son-in-law. "In autumn, I'll take you
and Carrie to the *Día de los Muertos* festival..." Isabel continued
to drone, skirting her central intent like always, following tan-
gents before arriving at some obscure point. Avra wished for
silence or a meditation session, when Isabel would chant *Om* on
an overstuffed pillow. Not this. Carrie seemed engrossed elsewhere, at least, in the circles of her cereal. Pushing O's with her
spoon, she watched them pop to the surface. Avra fought the
fear that Carrie would one day be ashamed of her, her injured
hand or some other part – reconstructed toes, or something not
even physical – enough to prefer Isabel as her primary family.
There weren't other alternatives; Stephen was gone and Sarah,
his sister in North Carolina, had made it clear that she didn't
have time for those he left behind. Avra barely knew her dead
grandmother's sister, Una, who was dying from Alzheimer's.

Una reminded her of Eva: her dead grandmother. Avra
hadn't thought of her in weeks. They'd spent five summers together, on the road for most of those months. Back then, Avra
had resented her grandmother's botanical bonanzas, wishing
that her dead mother might reappear magically to rescue her.
Avra never could have anticipated that her mother, one day,
would indeed magically reappear – but the "rescue" was ques-
tionable.

"...parade in the Mission District," Isabel continued. Avra tried to ignore her, washing the glass and letting the water run.

"...candied skulls with names across the foreheads..."

Avra fumbled with the faucet and glanced out the window. Fog laced the backyard. Nasturtium vines threaded calla lilies and artichoke plants (her mother's self-proclaimed "heart harvest"). In the corner of the garden, a crabapple tree littered the ground with small, inedible fruits. Branches dangled mirror-plated plastic birds.

"...mariachi bands, homemade floats and masks..."

Wanting to scream, Avra took a deep breath. She sensed a foreboding of what lay ahead, wanting to do everything for Carrie but unable to write her own name legibly, open cans and jars and do basic things. At least, she had managed to get a part-time job as a gallery guard at the Academy of Sciences.

A jingle from Beagle's collar announced Isabel's mutt. The dog wandered to Carrie's chair and sat.

"All dedicated to the spirits of the dead who return each year to rejoin loved ones. Sometimes you'll hear name-calling followed by the word *Presente!* as in, *his or her spirit is here!* Throughout Latin America, given hundreds of thousands of victims in civil wars – "

"What does this have to do with Stephen?" Avra interrupted, trying to keep her voice calm and restrained.

Isabel conducted her finger, as if visibly retracing the digression in her thought process. "Marigolds!" She stopped fidgeting. "Marigolds are the main flower used in the *Día*...you know. Altars in cemeteries and homes – "

Avra felt the weight of *The Street Enters the House* and started moving backwards.

"...burning copal. On the first *día* dedicated to children who have died, a path of petals is scattered for souls to find their way home." Isabel's fingers fluttered through the air, as if scattering invisible flowers. Avra felt movement in the absent extensions of her hand. "I was reminded of the festival because I used marigolds in this morning's *puja* for Stephen."

Avra rubbed her finger grafts. Her mother had made another *puja* elsewhere in the house to heal her hand injury. *Pujas* were a kind of daily worship based in Hindu tradition involving a shrine, Isabel had explained. For Avra's, she had arranged anatomical drawings, palmistry maps, poseable artists' models with hinged knuckles and joints. In every realm of Isabel's house, there was some altar or shrine: Hindu, Christian, Jewish, Muslim, Buddhist. Avra didn't know what derived from what, only that collectively they were devoted to remembering the dead, healing survivors, or appealing to gods. Tabletops held camphor-burning wick lamps, shallow bowls of flowers and crabapples from the yard, vessels with small spoons for sprinkling water over vermilion, turmeric, ash. The smell of incense permeated the house, except the garage, where vents allowed drafts to dilute heady fragrances.

"How can you?" asked Avra.

"What?"

Avra said nothing, just thought: *How can you mourn some-*

one you've never met? What right do you have?

Isabel slowly shook her head, smiling, making some un-spoken allowance. Avra tried not to feel disarmed by Isabel's at-tentions to the world's spiritual devotions but not, at least until recently, to her own family. It was as if, until Avra was physical-ly injured, she didn't fit into her mother's for-lack-of-a-better-word: cosmology. Was it a mindset? A conglomerate religion? There wasn't an easy classification for her mother's words and deeds, their origins and interrelations – except *How to Wear a Habit,* the name of Isabel's store. The business was cross-list-ed in the Yellow Pages under *Religious Organizations* and *Travel,* geared to those planning visits to countries with nationalized religions, or to communities so steeped in sacred influence that entering the culture obliged some attention to spiritual prac-tices and traditions. Avra had visited the shop in the Fillmore District and perused its dizzying array of rosaries, prayer rugs, menorahs, burkas, and calendar of events, forums and eve-ning lectures, sponsored by local mosques, churches, temples, and synagogues. "For people seeking to broaden their outlook on faith," Isabel had explained. Avra considered her mother's track record, watching the sarong's dancing hemline. She knew too well that Isabel might yet undergo another metamorpho-sis – and it might not involve her daughter and granddaughter.

Avra turned to go downstairs, but Carrie gasped. "God's in my cereal!"

Avra paled. *What kind of mother am I?*

"Where?" asked Isabel slowly, resting her teacup on the

table, peering over the bowl, calling Carrie by nickname, "*Mariposa*, show me God in your cereal."

Avra was stupefied, speechless, able to think only of words she'd read somewhere, *If you have formed a Circle to go into, Go into it yourself & see how you would do*. She didn't know whether to laugh, cry, or show no emotion. Her father would have retreated to the nearest turntable and turned up the volume, loud enough so she'd feel music inside her, or inside the music, resonance in her blood and bones. She wished he were here and said meekly, "Carrie, why did you say that?"

"Nana...?" Carrie looked inquisitively at her grandmother, while scooping up one of the grain-baked circles in a pool of milk, then swallowing.

"Look," said Isabel.

Avra peered back at the willow bowl.

"Not there." Isabel pointed out the window into the garden. Avra cautiously peered at tangles of orange and yellow petals, rustling against gray. Fog made everything appear spectral. Some vines blew upward, waving freely, until the tendrils touched, almost completing a circle.

"Without beginning, without end," said Isabel.

The vines fell to the ground.

"The end," Avra exhaled, realizing that she was holding her breath again. Her mother semi-bowed, pressing her palms in front of her chest, extending her body into a yoga pose. *Was it yoga or some cult? What was all this?*, Avra wondered, pinching herself to make sure she wasn't in a nightmare.

"Try this," Isabel said, coiling her arms together, then standing flamingo-like, curling one leg around the other.

"I can!" said Carrie, standing, imitating her grandmother's pose. Avra looked at the perched pair. Carrie seemed increasingly comfortable, despite frequent nightmares. How could Avra prevent her from following Isabel's footsteps? Isabel's eccentricity and unusual intelligence might also have endeared Avra – if Isabel were someone else's mother.

"Good for you," Avra said, hard-pressed to criticize, given her free housing. Her head ached. When Carrie laughed with Isabel, the kitchen seemed to deflate.

"Manuel's coming to dinner," Isabel said, straightening and gliding back toward the counter. The sarong fell into place without needing readjustment.

"I screeeaaaaam!" shrilled Carrie.

Avra winced.

"I'm sure Manuel will bring *ice cream*," corrected Isabel. Manuel was Isabel's boyfriend of two years and made a point to bring home-churned iced ginger, green tea, bean paste. At least, Avra thought, Isabel would be calmer with Manuel. He, too, had immersed in monastic life and was now "merging his old and new selves" in a more social sphere. At age 39, he was eight years Isabel's junior, a decade older than Avra, earning his living as a Bikram yoga instructor and training in a kind of calligraphic painting called *bokuseki* ("ink traces," he had translated). His original profession had been computer programming, but recovery from prostate cancer had prompted

a two-year training at a center in Marin County to become a
Zen monk. He'd written a book about the experience and given
a public reading at the store – one thing, then another, and he
became Isabel's de facto consultant on technological matters
for the shop, line of books and website: www.wearahabit.com.

The weight of the *The Street Enters the House* finally over-
whelmed Avra. "I'll be right back." She left the room before
Isabel could say a word.

The stairwell was dark, since the bulb had been removed.
Avra couldn't see painted saints, sculpted skulls, and feathered
masks, but felt their hazy gazes. The ground floor was cold. Instead of entering her makeshift space in the garage, she went
to Carrie's room.

The room seemed brighter than usual, lit from a full
moon, a rare exposure. Avra walked straight to the bookcase,
and urged *The Street Enters the House* onto a shelf. Beagle followed
and flopped at her feet. The book fell open, but Avra didn't read
the words. Nor did she turn to the closet, filled with odds and
ends, including Stephen's ashes. Instead, her attention focused
on her daughter's totems, almost all of them from Isabel: a toy
ark with animals, a statue of Ganesha, a shofar. Beside the religious items, cardboard boxes held vegetable-shaped beads,
alphabet dice, and pierced shells. With her good hand, Avra
reached for an ear of corn whose tiny husks bent into a heart-
shaped loop.

She returned the cob to its box. But as she pulled away,
the container slipped. Tiny cubes clapped against the floor.

Awkwardly trying to catch others as they fell, she knocked down the alphabet dice. A's, U's, and M's. H and A landed adjacently, HA – an untimely joke. Glancing to make sure the noise hadn't disturbed Beagle, Avra knelt, scooped the dispersed letters, and returned them to their shelf above polished stones. Her eyes began to glaze, blinking back tears.

She couldn't manage to keep beads in their boxes. She had lost touch with her life, including former friends, her photography, her teaching. Avra didn't have much of anything, except necessities, and focused on relearning to dress herself, to get a job that didn't involve her hand, to get Carrie adjusted to their new life, to cope with the loss of Stephen.

Yearning for some kind of comfort, or escape, she feared pity: wide-eyed sympathetic gazes, or worse, presumptuous condolences like: *I know how you feel.*

The bookcase started to blur: the alphabet, shrunken animals, plastic fruits, shells. She brushed her eyes with her sleeve and focused on gems. The rock samples were small, affixed to styrofoam in cardboard boxes printed with dual classifications: scientific and common names. Lustery gray *hematite*, glassy black *obsidian*, striped *zebra marble*. Larger samples filled a bigger box and included descriptions. She picked up a little card beside one chunk: "Dendrite," it read, "is a tree-shaped mineral that crystallizes onto another through a fractured edge of rock, resembles a fossilized fern or plant, and is collected for the interesting scenes it creates."

She tasted salt on her lips, more tears. More slid down her

cheeks; she wiped her eyes with the back of her hand. The tears fell silently; there was no heaving or sobbing. She felt empty. A wave swept over her, recurring often since Stephen's death, this feeling that went beyond grief, to nothing.

Except Carrie.

She had to keep going for their daughter, to help her cope with these changes. Looking for some direction, Avra scanned the bottom of the bookcase: *Karst Geomorphology and Hydrology, Underground Water Tracing, The Natural History of Biospeleology.* The books had been Stephen's, from his university carrel, but now were hers. An arbitrary inheritance, like her father had bequeathed opera librettos, 78s and 45s, after years of collecting. He'd taken them everywhere, as they'd moved from military base to base, and never settled long enough in one place. More than in apartments, Avra had felt most at home when her father retreated to his records, hummed or sang along. Although she'd rebelled against his hope for her to be a musician, if someone had asked where home was, she'd be pressed to admit it was music: *Spem in alium, Messe en Si Mineur, Les Noces.* In her mind, harmonies surfaced under titles on the bookshelf: *Growth Banding in Stalagmites and Stalactites, Geomicrobiology, Cave Life: Evolution and Ecology.* Her father had taught her to listen for music anywhere, since he'd raised Avra alone. Their only times apart had been summers when Avra visited Eva in Oregon. His records and librettos had gathered dust in boxes after his death, after Avra moved around the country, turned to photography and, with Stephen, started descending into subterranean caves. *Carbonates and Evaporites, Fractal Dimensions and Geometries of Caves, To Photograph Darkness—.*

She'd started photographing at night and underground, when they went caving. *To Photograph Darkness* was the last book Stephen had given her. Or almost given, since it was found in his office desk wrapped for her birthday, and inscribed under the subtitle *The History of Underground and Flash Photography*: "To Avra – everything that you are and will be." She couldn't manage to hold a camera and equipment now, and hadn't read the book, which was relegated to Carrie's shelves like all books from Stephen's office carrel, except those claimed by friends in his department.

It was still there, waiting.

Hesitating, she reached out her left hand. Awkwardly, she slid the book off the shelf, propped it open to a random page. Inside, figures were faceless; gauzy textures made them ghost-like. A sepia-toned picture revealed the difficulty of early exposures, when a sitter had to remain unmoving for minutes in front of an open lens' shutter, when photographs were believed to steal a subject's soul. The only focused object was a sarcophagus, behind the blurred foreground. "Inside the Great Pyramid, Giza," the caption listed the Grand Gallery, Queen's Chamber, King's Chamber, "the celebrated 'coffer' was photographed from a variety of positions..."

Avra stopped reading and left the book, feeling vacant again. This wasn't what she needed. Maybe in another time or place, she might've studied the images or considered photographic capabilities, or felt something symphonic in relations between light and darkness. No longer. She lifted her left hand, like a badge of her partiality, stared at it and imagined that if she looked long enough – more closely than anything she'd scrutinized – the fingers might grow back. Her toes, too. But she'd been rearranged, unexpectedly, not the hip bone connected to the femur, but phalanges from her toes to her knuckles. She'd been assured that a person can be reconstructed and survive. Breasts were reconstructed by moving tissue from a buttocks or elsewhere to reconstruct a chest; and hadn't she heard of a plastic surgeon who'd devised a way to make wings? She wanted none of that. If Isabel hadn't insisted on the surgery, she would've gotten a prosthesis, at most.

Beagle nudged her. Avra felt herself smile, a foreign feeling. Petting him with the flat of her hand prompted a low moan, almost purring. As her hand moved over his fur, she missed something much more than her fingers, and wished that Carrie would remember Stephen. They talked so seldom about him, unless Avra brought him up; then Carrie's mind would drift to a friend at school or a coveted toy, and leave Avra's throat lodged with words.

Straightening up, she noticed *The Street Enters the House* opened on the edge of the shelf. A few words caught her attention: skimmed a column of trilogies, paused and listened (before she left the book and headed to her makeshift room, to change for dinner, while:) water continued to wash roads and meadows, and he noticed a solitary cow. As the train speedily approached and passed, he pressed his nose to the glass to see the black-and-white bovine lift its head from the ground and gnaw, making the man's mind regurgitate reticulum, abomasum, omasum, and rumen, like cud in the four chambers of the holstein's stomach. Arturo considered the crushed mush akin to *wet wheat*, which made him forget the cow and recall his newest concoction, a milky-way of stars and strings and super strings. And it became **the next subject** drawn in his notebook.

Looking at the sketch, he noticed an arced noodle, as associations roamed and revolved and retreated into remote recesses that **stirred more thoughts**, coagulating and branching as easily as neurons stimulate dentrites and axons; as scribbling stirred more ingredients into his and Nova's scheme; as he conceived new recipes for their hypothetical restaurant. Under anise eyes, the smile floated, **taunting** him to circumscribe it, and add a stem. A jack-o-lantern emerged, and Arturo thought of masks he was bringing to Nova and his one-year-old son, Simon. Halloween was Nova's favorite holiday, four days away, so Arturo had spent the morning at a toystore to surprise her with a stash of fuzzy muzzles. He was pleased with the **textures** of the costume faces – the plastic noses, wire whiskers, fur that varied in length around ears, brows, snouts, and megaphone mouths: of a leopard, lion, and she-wolf. He had wanted to buy a lion, tiger, and bear because Simon was transfixed by a picture-book by Baum and ran around the house gurgling *zo, zo, nam nit, ot ot!*, like his parents reversed the story's **syllables** when they narrated it to him at bedtime – but no. At the toystore, Mr. Alabaster had said *out-of-stock*. The toyman suggested an equally tactilic trio and, in consolation, gave Arturo a wind-up tiger. *Would she want to write of...?* Arturo thought of options as he sat in the train, remembering the artificial zoo. He put pad and pen in his pocket and reached under the seat.

From that berth, he retrieved a paper sac that crinkled as it opened, as he dug **into the contents**. Soft fuzz, plastic knobs, wiry wisps – each texture rolled masks through Arturo's mind. Mr. Alabaster had taken time to find the best masks by **shuffling** through the basement: through stray puzzle pieces, **tangled** mobiles, wings off model planes, chipped marbles, gyroscopes sans string, single *Menschenalphabeten*. Distracted, the toyman had cranked a jack-in-the-box, then opened a magician's chest with a secret door to hide *a shell for a pen, a magnet for a stone*. *Dimestore alchemy*, he chimed, as **sounds** of the store whirled *cheep cheep, mulberry, waddy, give your purr a plink* in Arturo's ears again, in the train, as he unwrapped a parcel, pulled out Tabitha, squinted at the tiger, and recalled how to wind her.

Unclamping the battery holder, Arturo swung open her belly to discover a compartment marked + and -. Circuits and currents charged Arturo's mind with particles that attracted, repelled and flowed volts, joules, amps, columbs, and ohms. Tabitha's eyes opened, shunted left and right, her ears bent **forward, back** and after eight steps a pink tongue spit from her mouth, groveling: *Groar.*

Groar, groar, Tabitha said again, in the train.

As the tiger rolled her eyes and popped her tongue, the woman in the adjacent seat didn't acknowledge Arturo's or the tiger's presence, only her book. Arturo glimpsed her emerald ring tracing phrases, on a page half-filled with text. Her hand stopped. Fingers slipped down the spine to *yes I said yes I will*

—Tickets?, a voice grumbled.

The novel speaks! Arturo thought and leaned closer to the woman's lap to hear.

—Mister? Up here, I don't have all day, the voice grumbled again.

Arturo turned his face toward the man with a slateblue cap that matched his uniform.

—Tickets?, the conductor groaned and held up his fist of stubs.

The woman reached into the front cover of her book, closing the page of *yeses*, and removed a slip of paper that the conductor considered feasible proof of her transport. He ignored her and focused on Arturo, who sat clutching the toy tiger. ...*ch, ch, ch*... Tabitha's plastic backlegs scraped in their joints as she walked on air, crossed her eyes, and lolled her tongue like clockwork.

—Mister?, the conductor swelled.

Groar. Grrr.... Tabitha stopped squirming and mewling.

Arturo retrieved and handed his stub. The conductor tore the perforation, as the velour woman smiled.

The rain had stopped. Sky spread with clumps of yellow-orange tinged without storm-gray. Arturo almost admired the **colorful contortions**, clouds, clouds...like caves, faults, stalactites, centripedals, trelliseds...drainage **patterns** offered ideas to represent condensation, precipitation, and occlusion...why not clouds, to complement their meals-to-feel?

As Arturo chewed on notions, an inventory started spilling,

slippery boiled eggs and soft airy loaves dipped, to chew and ex-hale like smoking snow. "Clouding," he formulated a subdefinition beside "making opaque or ominous," is "puffing produced from the intake of edible substances dipped in liquid nitrogen, whose freeze contacts a warm mouth like breath against winter's chill, and emits mist as cirrus, cumulus, nimbus, or stratus." He couldn't predict the cloud-kind until he tried to cook. **As experiment –**

Experiments – all his efforts were procedures carried out un-der controlled conditions to un-cover unknown effects or laws, to re-cover what was presumed lost and what lay **shrouded** like a land-scape in a storm that drenched a train, as it slithered rickety crack-ity thrum, which could lull a body to sleep or entice a mind to spin sugar in webs a dozen inches tall-and-wide, which wound round to hide the innermost ingredient, a solitary tapioca truffle filled with pudding & a fleshy litchi: the heart of that dish.

Yes, Arturo thought as the train hummed, *our diners must un-ravel the web to get to the heart of the dish. If we can lead to the heart, whose center isn't easily held, if we can serve the senses, split like atoms before they slip, if I, if Nova – if we can orbit the essence then maybe possibly. Hopefully, doubtfully veritably charitably sin-fully mercifully faithlessly faithfully what was lost, may be regained.*

Now all they had to do was open the restaurant, and stop planning. But there was always one more idea to render. "The Storm, the Fly, & the Heart." Arturo dug his notebook out of his pocket and sketched the heart, which suddenly on the page began to ("...help?" Manuel said.

Looking up from re-reading, Avra said, "What?" She was

tired after a long shift at the museum and wanted only to be left alone.

"Did it help?" he asked again. His voice was kind and soft. Two days earlier, he had offered to disassemble *The Street Enters the House* into sections: manageably-sized paperbacks. Patiently, now, he stood in his untucked shirt and loose pants, shaved head and sandals. His gentle manner put her at ease.

"Yes," she replied.

"I thought this might, too." Manuel slowly lifted up an old laptop computer. He handled the laptop calmly. Everything about Manuel seemed to occur in slow motion. "I rebuilt this from recycled parts." He put down the computer, went to the hallway, and brought back a card table.

Avra didn't want another handout. Isabel had taken out second mortgages on the house and store to finance her hand operation. As if the fire hadn't been bad enough, Avra's health insurance had expired shortly before that happened. *Needlessly*, Avra thought, feeling the unwanted debt. She would be paying back her mother forever.

"This is from me – not Isabel," Manuel said, as if reading her mind. "I installed a processor that's fast enough to support voice-activated software."

Within minutes, the screen glowed from a multi-colored encircled square, rimmed with flame-like figures, bursting with thunderbolts and petals.

"There she is," he said, pointing at the screen. "The logo for voice-recognition looks like a shaggy beast – can you see the software icon against the mandala screensaver?" He pointed, and Avra squinted to distinguish it from the intricate design.

Isabel popped her head in the doorway, "I'll put Carrie to bed and steep some tea."

She was gone before Avra or Manuel could respond.

"The icon corresponds with the name of the software, *Speaking to the Sphinx*. Click the image, and boxed commands will prompt you through the training session, then you'll be ready to write whatever you want." He watched Avra's blank expression. "Don't think too hard about this. You only need to train the system. Basically, the program receives sound waves of your voice, which vary in length and translate into different mathematical algorithms. The drive stores these as memory to match similar sequences when they're transmitted again – so, the program learns to recognize individual voices."

Avra had never heard Manuel say so many words.

"Don't worry about the mechanics," he said. "The important thing is that it works, more or less. You'll see where it falls short. But technology continues to improve. A few years ago, this existed only in the realm of imagination."

"Almost done?" Isabel called from upstairs.

"You should start the training," said Manuel.

"I'm going to pass on tea," said Avra.

He turned to go.

She stood. "Thanks."

"We give what we can."

She did a double-take, thinking of his words. His feet padded up the stairs, then his voice commingled with Isabel's, chanting meditatively. Avra left the computer and walked down the hall to Carrie's room. She lay on the floor in pajamas, smiling under glow-in-the-dark stars with outstretched arms, swaying clenched hands.

"Are you flying?" Avra asked.

Carrie dropped her arms, tilting back her head to see her mother. "The animals are." She unclenched her fingers.

"I think the animals are tired. Why don't we put them to bed?"

"They're not tired."

I'm tired, Avra thought but didn't say. "A story?"

"Wizard!" Carrie rolled into a ball, onto her knees and sprang to her feet, still clasping the animals in her hands. She transferred the trio to the bookcase and pulled out a worn text. *Oz* was the last story Avra wanted to read, but it had become Carrie's favorite since all the characters followed the Yellow Brick Road to awake from their nightmare. *I might as well get it over for tonight*, Avra thought and joined Carrie on the bed.

"What chapter did we end with last time?" asked Avra.

"The Scarecrow and Dorothy found the house in the forest."

Avra knew the place and thumbed through pages until she arrived at Chapter V: "The Rescue of the Tin Woodman." Reclining against pillows, she began to narrate with different voices for the characters. Carrie watched intensely. Page after page. After a black-and-white woodcut showed the travelers meeting the paralyzed metal man, a watercolored golden path prompted Carrie to sing, "Follow, follow, follow!" repeatedly, because she didn't know other lyrics. A few pages later, Avra was relieved to see white space that marked the end of the chapter.

"The end. For tonight." She swung her legs off the bed and started to stand.

"More!" Carrie pulled her arm.

"Imagine a field of poppies, and go to sleep." Avra smoothed the comforter, then her daughter's bangs.

"I'm not tired." She started bouncing. *"Humpty dumpty sat on a wall, Humpty dumpty had a great fall!"* She tumbled to the floor, laughing, wiggling her legs and arms.

"Carrie!" Avra sighed, unable to scoop up the spider-like limbs. "Sometimes when you're not sleepy, you still have to go to bed."

Carrie sat up with a jolt. "Let's sing *Do, Re, Mi!*"

"Enough for tonight. Tomorrow." Avra sat on the edge of the bed. Carrie begrudgingly returned and tucked herself under the covers. Avra kissed her forehead, walked to the doorway and turned out the light. "Sweet dreams."

"Promise?"

"Promise?" Avra turned abruptly, thinking Carrie was asking her to pledge the quality of her dreams.

"Tomorrow night?" pleaded her daughter.

"Yes. *Do, Re, Mi* tomorrow night."

"Another chapter? Singing? Both?"

"We'll see." Despite the darkness, she saw Carrie's index and middle fingers glide almost automatically into her mouth. "What did we say about sucking fingers? Nana will have to paint your nails with sour polish again."

Carrie's hands slipped out of her mouth. "No!"

"She won't, if your fingers stay out of your mouth. Come on." Avra pulled them out, as always, to make her daughter curb the habit. No movements of Avra's left hand felt like habit. Every gesture felt foreign, as if she were trapped in a stranger's body. Carrie hid her hands under the covers. "That's my girl," Avra said. "Good night."

In the hallway, the monotone of Isabel and Manuel drifted from upstairs. Avra tiptoed to the garage, toward a glow whose source she didn't recognize at first, until she stood in the doorframe. Instead of turning the computer off, she sat on the edge of the mattress, kicked off Velcro shoes, and reclined on pillows before rummaging for pajamas. None of her old clothes had survived the fire; anything new was chosen for minimal hand use. Few or no buttons or ties. Pullovers, elasticized waists, and Velcro fasteners. Finding an old pullover robe from Isabel, she thought the wing-like sleeves and cowl appeared like a nun's habit. The irony almost made her laugh. She laughed at what she was trying to manage. At least, her thumb remained. Microsurgery had attached functioning nerves, muscles, and veins of the grafted toes to two phalanges on her knuckles; fine motor skills and tactile training were part of the protocol for her physical therapy program. Sometimes, she could feel sensations in her

absent fingers; her doctor had reassured her that this was usual, and there was biological basis for amputees' experiences of
phantom limbs and physiological memories (*and people?* she'd
wanted to ask. *Is there biological basis for feeling phantom people?*).
The doctor had shown her a map of the parietal lobes and the
relatively large receptor regions for hands compared to other
areas of the body. "Some areas are more sensitive than others,"
he'd said, "and receive input every moment. That input is then
evaluated in the brain, a living organism that constantly maps
and remaps the body's functions according to an intricate relay
of feedback; and extrinsic trauma can disrupt..." *Enough,* Avra
told herself. She wished she didn't have a talent for remembering. Forgetfulness would be a gift.

Wearing the habit-like robe, she walked to the computer
and sat, picked up the headset microphone, adjusted its band
awkwardly, with the foam-covered recorder in front of her
mouth. Her left hand remained in her lap. She moved her right
hand to the touchpad, sliding her fingers, so the screen's arrow
landed on the Sphinx.

A box popped up with the words *New Participant* on the
toolbar, which was then covered by a second box, headed *Training the Sphinx.*

*Welcome! You will be asked to read a sentence aloud. When
you're ready, click Proceed.*

She clicked *Proceed.*

A new sentence appeared in the box-within-a-box. She
read aloud: "In this brave new world of continuous speech rec-

ognition, you will learn to speak clearly and articulately to the Sphinx. As you follow...."

From the lingo, she already doubted the program. Brave New World? Sphinx? Classics as jargon. The yellow arrow turned red to prompt her to speak. "As you follow," she proceeded through the instructions.

"Who are you talking to?" she heard from behind. Avra turned and saw Carrie standing in the doorway, rubbing her eyes.

"You're supposed to be asleep."

"I'm not tired. Who are you talking to?" Carrie wandered into the room and gazed at the screen. The arrow flashed red. Since moving in with Isabel, Avra had begun to feel self-conscious around everyone, including her daughter. Trying not to sound as foolish as she felt, she said, "I was reading to the computer."

"You said no more reading tonight."

"This is a special computer that listens to Mommy's voice and writes down what she says. But it has to learn what Mommy sounds like. Like you can tell the difference between Nana and Mommy when we speak, even with your eyes closed." Avra had grown strangely accumstomed to referring to herself in the third person, at least with Carrie.

"No, I don't."

"But you can."

Carrie stared at the computer. "Does it talk to you?"

"It listens."

The girl scuttled close to the screen. "Who?" Her small

finger almost touched the Sphinx on the toolbar, beside smaller images of a microphone, a piece of paper, and a book with a questionmark on the cover.

"That," Avra said for lack of a better answer.

"What?"

"It's called a Sphinx."

Carrie touched the screen. Avra gently, partially, clasped her daughter's hand and said, "Careful. Don't touch." The small fingers curled over the groove between her thumb and grafts. *I guess I'm talking to the Sphinx*, Avra thought. *If only the Sphinx could answer.* "It's late. You should go to bed."

"NOoooooooooo," Carrie shrieked on the verge of a tantrum, gripping Avra's hand to the point of pinching. Then abruptly, her grasp relaxed; her voice diminished to a whisper. She sat up and folded her hands. "Please?"

Avra almost smiled at her daughter's self-restraint. She remembered when they'd first played hide-and-seek, Carrie would curl up in the middle of the floor in plain sight, cover her eyes and say, "I'm hiding, come and find me." It was exactly how Avra often felt. "If you stay, you have to be very quiet."

"Yes, yes." Carrie climbed into her lap, shifted for a few minutes, then laid her head against Avra's shoulder. Avra turned back toward the screen. *Reading Selections* listed a dozen-or-so excerpts, categorized parenthetically as *Literature, Science-fiction, Fairy Tale, Business Manual*. She looked for anything age-appropriate and noticed *Alice and the Looking Glass*. A new box opened, and a yellow arrow pointed to the first word, *Hold*. Remembering to read at a normal pace, slowly and articulately, she began: "'Hold *your* tongue!' cried the Tiger Lily. 'As if *you* ever saw....'"

She read about two-dozen paragraphs, not stopping because this initial exercise was recording her voice's speech waves, not translating dictation: "'..."nonsense" if you like,' she said, 'but *I've* heard nonsense, compared with which that would be as sensible as a dictionary!'"

A box opened on the screen and blocked the excerpt.

Congratulations! the new box read. *You've successfully finished your training session. Click Proceed, and the Sphinx will save your voice in its memory. If the Sphinx has trouble understanding you in the future, repeat the training session. You can always ask it questions by clicking the Help menu. In the meantime, in a few moments, you'll be ready to begin dictating.*

"Keep reading," said Carrie.

The Sphinx is going to bed now," Avra said. "And so must you, too."

Carrie nodded *no*, emphatically, and her bangs fell across her eyes. Avra brushed them aside with her right hand, tucked them behind her daughter's ear, and wondered about the source of her incessant energy. She began to disentangle Carrie's limbs from her lap. "Off we go."

Carrie wrestled to stay seated, pressing, "What happens to Alice?"

For a moment, Avra thought of Isabel's original name. "She has many adventures. We'll read the whole story sometime. But now – "

"Why is the queen red?"

"Carrie. She's the queen of hearts, and hearts are red."

"Why?"

Avra pushed her daughter gently off her lap. Carrie's feet shuffled in place, as she pointed again to the icon on the screen. "Bed, now," Avra said sternly. Carrie squirmed and fussed, tugging the sleeves of the robe. Avra felt suddenly exhausted, thinking of the hours ahead, trying to calm her daughter. Her glance fell on the only photograph of Stephen, smiling nonchalantly with a spelunker's hardhat, flashlight, belt of notebooks and sample vials – all slightly underexposed.

As Carrie kept fussing, Avra became angry, at the photograph, at Stephen, for coming into her life, for making her care, then for leaving her and Carrie alone, for everything that had spiraled out of sequence. It seemed like yesterday when he'd posed in the mouth of that cave, when everything had seemed as if it were meant to be, when she'd printed the picture inadequately, never anticipating what lay ahead.

After putting Carrie to bed and returning to her own room, Avra turned off the light. Recorded throat-singing, with buzzing and whistling overtones, wafted from upstairs. After counting sheep, mumbling lullabies, and trying to chant *Om*, nothing had induced her to sleep. Anxious and restless, she turned on the light and found a cut-out section of *The Street Enters the House* and flipped randomly, to what seemed like a second title page:

T   H   E
O
P   A   L   A   T   E
Y

by francamano
o
v
a

A *Table of Contents* unraveled thereafter, page after page, listing hundreds of fairy tales. Along the margin ran a quoted invocation: "Tell me a story. / In this century, and moment, of mania, / Tell me a story. / Make it a story of great distances, and starlight. / The name of the story will be..." Skimming through titles, Avra recognized *The Ugly Duckling, Snow White, Sleeping Beauty, The Tortoise & the Hare, The Giant who Hid his Heart Outside his Body*, and many others, until *Stone Soup* caught her eye. Slowly she flipped to that page, which looked like a play, with a cast of characters. But already her eyes felt heavy. Deciding to save the fairy tale for another day, she turned out the light and fell asleep.

INTERMISSION

(Mira gestorum)

Stone Soup;
or, a Recipe Plied with Plight

(A TRAGICOMEDY IN ONE ACT)

Characters

Narrator
First Soldier
Second Soldier
Third Soldier
Old Man
Old Woman
Well-Woman
Miranda
Assorted Townspeople (Boy, Grandmother, Foster
        Father, Postman, Farmer, Rabbi, Belly-Dancer,
        Shaman, Young Punk, Painter, Preacher, Doctor.
        Note: Numbered Townspeople can be divided
        among characters, or assigned to audience
        members.)

Setting / Time

A ghost town at a crossroads. Midday. Three closed doors face a road, scattered with stones. One stone is bigger than the rest.

NARRATOR

(*Narrator enters left and stands aside, reading an oversized children's book.*) Once upon a time, three Soldiers got hungry while returning from The War. (*Soldiers enter right.*) The Soldiers were considered "Enemies of the State," even though the State was their Homeland. All ranks and reasons had become confused. Without material possessions, the Soldiers were resourceful, at least enough to disbelieve whispers from cracked-open doors:

ALL

(*In unison, from behind doors.*) There is nothing.

NARRATOR

Other wayfarers might have left the crossroads, but one soldier spied a last cracked-open door and pled:

FIRST SOLDIER

A stone! Can you at least spare a stone?

NARRATOR

(*Door #2 opens slowly.*) An Old Man pointed to the littered path and muttered:

OLD MAN

(*Distrusting.*) Stones are for the taking. For what?

FIRST SOLDIER

For soup.

OLD MAN

What an idea, to make soup from a stone.

NARRATOR

And, thus, the first ingredient was procured: by whim and because it seemed negligible. Scooping up a stone by the Old Man's door, the First Soldier stood with his compatriots and considered its culinary potential. The Old Man's wife popped her head from the house.

OLD WOMAN

(*Coming through same door, rubbing hands in her apron.*) What's this all about?

OLD MAN

(*Scratching his beard.*) These soldiers think they can make soup from a stone.

WELL-WOMAN

(*Off-stage as if her cry comes from nowhere.*) Don't go outside!

SECOND SOLDIER

(*Glancing slowly left to right.*) Where is that voice coming from?

OLD WOMAN

(*Laughing nervously.*) What an idea—to make soup from a stone! You might as well try to make wine from a well. We don't consider that kind of nonsense here. We're practical people. Anyways, you can't make soup without a kettle.

SECOND SOLDIER

A kettle would greatly help.

OLD WOMAN

(*Hesitating.*) I have such a pot. (*Turning to her husband.*)
Father, please go and fetch it. (*Exit Old Man through their door.*
Old Woman shakes her head.) What an idea, to make soup from
a...

WELL-WOMAN

(*Off-stage.*) Soup from a stone? Soup from a stone?

NARRATOR

The gathering looked toward a barely-opened window of a
neighbor's house. A young woman's face appeared.

WELL-WOMAN

(*Opens and exits Door #1, holding up an empty picture*
frame, looking through.) Soup from a stone? Soup is slurped by
spoon, and you can't spoon a stone, like you can't tune a moan.
(*Second Soldier makes a deferential bow. Old Woman shakes her*
head. Well-Woman listens and blushes, flirtingly.) That was nothing. What you need is water, and I have a well. It's out back;
there's no lack. If the Farmer gives fodder, you're welcome to
my water. (*Well-Woman waves her arm to enter her door, and*
Second Soldier follows.) Come, come in. You fetch a pail, and
I'll tell you a tale.

OLD MAN

(*Returning through Door #2, lugging large kettle.*) Ow, ow, ow! (*Townspeople look toward Old Man, who drags kettle down his path, pushes it upright, and grunts.*) That was a chore and worked up my appetite. (*Looking skeptically at Soldiers.*) If you do make this so-called Stone Soup, you must promise me the first bowl.

THIRD SOLDIER

(*Nodding.*) Of course! Of course! (*Well-Woman shrieks with laughter from off-stage.*)

THIRD SOLDIER

(*Slightly distracted, glancing toward Door #1.*) Once water arrives, we'll need to build a fire. Do you have wood? Newspapers? Matches?

OLD MAN

There's no shortage of wood. We have newspapers that no one wants because they're outdated. In my son's lean-to... (*He stops speaking. Old Woman turns away and hides her face in her hands. Old Man goes to her, wraps her in his arms, and lulls:*) Mother, mother... (*A palpable silence settles. Unpeeling his embrace, Old Man faces the bystanders.*) I will get a cord because we'll need a big fire to heat the big pot. (*He walks down the road stoically, while Second Soldier and Well-Woman spill out of her house, laughing. All eyes follow their motions.*)

WELL-WOMAN

(*Giggling and ogling Second Soldier.*) We're making soup from a stone, not hoarding something of our own! (*Second Soldier winks at her and at the other soldiers, then carries the splashing bucket to the kettle.*)

OLD WOMAN

(*Dabbing tears from her cheek with the edge of her apron.*)
Thyme, thyme. I almost forgot the ingredient that I add to everything, even pies. It has been my secret. If we use only water and a
stone, I don't trust there will be enough spice. (*Exit Old Woman.*)

WELL-WOMAN

(*Drifts to Second Soldier and asks with widening eyes:*)
How did you learn to make soup from a stone, not from sticks
or a bone?

SECOND SOLDIER

It's an old family recipe, passed down through generations.

WELL-WOMAN

Whose family? On whose side?

OLD MAN

(*Re-entering, huffing and puffing.*) Oh, oh, oh... (*Everyone's attention turns to Old Man, who cradles logs and kindling.*)
If one of you soldiers runs to the abandoned house down there,
you'll find a stack of newspapers on the porch. (*Third Soldier
takes his cue and returns with an armful, stuffs newsprint among
the logs, and lights the pile.*)

NARRATOR

Once the fire was flaming, the soup began to cook. And it
cooked. And it cooked. (*Enter more Townspeople, casually and
curiously.*) And it cooked. And it cooked. And it cooked. In the
hours that followed, villagers emerged cautiously from their
houses, peeping and creeping out of the woodworks.

BOY

(*Coming out of Door #3, pulling arm of Grandmother, who uses a cane.*) What smells so tasty?

NARRATOR

The villagers approached the cauldron in curiosity. They didn't come empty-handed but bore a little of *this*, of that— (*Postman interrupts:* "You can't use that alone!")—they said, throwing in each offering to make more than itself. (*Grandmother gestures to Postman to lift Boy above the pot's lip.*)

BOY

(*Smelling.*) Ooh, aah, oh!

NARRATOR

The boy saw bubbling shapes, colors, textures. He couldn't recognize most ingredients, from unfamiliar cuisines. Villagers had scrounged contributions from their pantries, cellars, secret storehouses. There were too many spices to name, excluding the Old Woman's thyme. The First Soldier removed a notebook from a sack that matched his fatigues.

FIRST SOLDIER

(*Holding out notebook.*) Whatever you bring, you must describe in this ledger. This will be a guide if someone needs to make Stone Soup again.

NARRATOR

The villagers lined up by the ledger and began to write, one by one. (*Townspeople proceed, murmuring in anticipation. Enter Miranda, riding toy pony with bulging saddlebags.*)

MIRANDA

Can the soup use more than a single stone?

NARRATOR

The Soldiers turned toward Miranda, who stood beside a
small burro with saddlebags.

THIRD SOLDIER

Why, surely, every contribution makes a difference!

NARRATOR

(*Miranda reaches into her saddlebag.*) As Miranda turned
toward her burro, the Soldiers noticed that her left hand was
missing. Her right hand pulled out a stone and cast it over the
brim. (*Miranda throws.*) Plop!, it splashed. She brushed her only
hand against her torn dress and said matter-of-factly:

MIRANDA

That was my Pet Rock, Sisyphus.

FIRST SOLDIER

(*Eyes widening.*) Sisyphus?

MIRANDA

(*Gesturing to her pony.*) Yes. And this is my burro, Dapple.
I collect stones. I have pebbles from an abandoned fish tank,
mini-replicas of Stonehenge and Mount Rushmore, a peach
pit—since it says in the dictionary that drupaceous fruits have
stones—and other Pet Rocks named Anaximander and Heracli-
tus. I have pictures of ancient Chinese Scholars Rocks and the
Omphalos Stone, which was considered the world's navel in its

day, and a postcard of giant carved faces on Easter Island. Nobody understands why the faces were carved or how they moved
from the middle of the island to the shoreline, but it's believed
they're deceased ancestors of the carvers, maybe even gods.
There's an astrolabe in my kit to make another stone, plus....
(*All start to move in slow motion, as Miranda mouths words in
silence. All listen and react with heightened gestures and facial
expressions, amused and slightly awed, before the play's action
speeds back to normal.*) ...an Egyptian scarab beetle inscribed
with chapter 30B of the Book of the Dead, which was laid on a
mummy's chest to prevent the heart from disclosing any earthly
misdemeanors of the deceased during the final judgment. I also
have a paper torn out of a book by my imaginary friend—she
knows I like stones and acts as my second pair of eyes—that
says: "The stones would cry out to testify." And my favorite
Grimm tale called *The Girl Without Hands* includes a king who
weeps that "a heavy stone has fallen from off my heart" after he
returns from a long journey and learns that the queen's hands,
which were chopped before he met her, have regrown; and she
no longer needs the silver hands he made her, which she keeps in
the inner room of her enforested house whose sign reads "Here
all dwell free"....

FOSTER FATHER

(*Huffing and puffing like he's blown down a house.*) Miranda! (*All eyes turn toward Foster Father.*)

NARRATOR

It was her father—a foster (but not a very nice one, unlike
many other fosters). Her real parents were Missing-in-Action.

FOSTER FATHER

(*Visibly angry.*) That's enough! Get back in the house. I
told you not to talk to strangers.

MIRANDA

(*Looking anxiously to each soldier.*) Please, please...

WELL-WOMAN

(*Hollering at Foster Father.*) No harm here! No fear!

FOSTER FATHER

(*Still panting.*) You...never...I...

MIRANDA

(*Looking desperately toward Soldiers.*) I want to be a stone-carver!

FOSTER FATHER

How many times do I have to tell you... (*Sighing, less mad than sad.*) You can't always have what you want.

WELL-WOMAN

No harm—no fear—

THIRD SOLDIER

Stone carving is a noble profession.

MIRANDA

(*Pausing to look back at Foster Father, then down at her missing hand, then at Soldiers.*) You think so? Even though I am what I am? (*Soldiers nod. Her clenched brow relaxes; her lips broaden into a grin.*) There are so many beautiful types: travertine, marble, limestone. I want to study lithology and learn the properties of each—some are harder than others and more supporting for columns, arches, and buttresses. Once the Materials

Board removes the mandate of metal for weapons, I plan to use steel with stones, for reinforcement. In the meantime, I carve tombstones, and make a lithograph now and then. (*Miranda looks hesitantly again from Soldiers to her Foster Father, who shakes his head and throws up his arms. Near the wings, Young Punk starts to fuss, spit, stir.*)

FIRST SOLDIER

Tell us more.

MIRANDA

(*Swallowing, standing taller.*) In my view, stones are our most core material but aren't appreciated because of their abundance. Remember Pyrrha and Deucalion, who considered stones to be their mother's bones, who threw them to repopulate the ravaged earth? If the universe had evolved differently, proportions of elements would've differed and then gold might be plentiful, and stones rare. And if this were true, then we might be making Gold Soup. (*Old Woman chuckles, exchanging a glance with Old Man. First Soldier tilts his head, thoughtfully. Third Soldier winks at Miranda, who grins.*) If you'd like, I'll put my scarab in the soup, so long as I get it back after the meal.

YOUNG PUNK

(*Pushing through crowd.*) Add *more* stones?! Stone soup— what a crock. I'll put you between a rock and a hard place. (*Makes fisticuffs.*) What are your intentions? For this soup and all of us?

WELL-WOMAN

Soup from a stone makes love on loan! (*No one pays attention. First Soldier gestures to Miranda to add more rocks.*)

YOUNG PUNK

(*Kicks dirt, like a bull preparing to charge. Boy backs slowly down the street, then rushes offstage. Townspeople ring Young Punk, who taunts:*) Stone Soup?! Stone Soup?! You think a recipe is gonna save us? (*First Soldier holds up ledger. As if blinded, Young Punk shrinks away, covering his face and hitting himself.*) What the...? (*ready to say "Fuck," but this is a PG play*)

OLD MAN

(*Stepping forward to face Young Punk.*) Enough! (*First Soldier draws the ledger back to his chest. Young Punk drops his fists, dazed as if unable to see.*) Where were you when my son needed... (*His voice trails off.*) Where were you when *we* needed you? (*Young Punk focuses to meet Old Man's stare, listening.*) Now, let the Soldier finish what he's trying to say.

OLD WOMAN

(*A bit flustered, gesturing toward the kettle.*) Would you look at that...

NARRATOR

The big black cauldron bubbled at the brim. Everyone scuttled toward the kettle.

BOY

(*To Grandmother.*) Can I taste it, can I?

GRANDMOTHER

May you. And say "please."

BOY

(*Articulating carefully.*) May I *please* taste the stone soup?

OLD WOMAN

I'll run inside and get a ladle. Father... (*Turning to Old Man.*) Go and fetch your toadstool. (*Both run into Door #2 and reemerge with ladle and toadstool.*)

BOY

(*Grandmother takes ladle, steps on stool, and scoops soup into Boy's small spoon. He tastes.*) Mmmm! My cocoa made the difference! And who added the parmesan? That's my favorite! (*Boy resubmerges his spoon in the big dipper and swallows again.*)

NARRATOR

The Soldiers smiled at the secret of the soup, while the townspeople scattered to their homes to retrieve odds and ends of bowls and utensils, returning for servings. One by one, each villager approached the kettle and filled their bowls. They stood around eating. With each spoonful or sip, they commented on discerned flavors.

FARMER

(*Adjusting his artificial leg.*) Oh, my persimmons!

PAINTER

What colors! What textures! What fragrance!

POSTMAN

(*Tipping cap.*) My pickle packed just enough dill.

RABBI

Horseradish balances against too much sweetness.

BELLY-DANCER

(*Jangling her skirt.*) Rasas make life relished!

SHAMAN

(*Puffing on a pipe.*) It's all in the roots. It's all in the roots. It's all in the roots.

OLD MAN

(*Turning to his wife.*) If I do say so myself, my wife's pot allowed all the ingredients to cook together.

OLD WOMAN

(*Blushing.*) No, hush now. We're just fortunate that the ingredients made so much. We'll have leftovers for days to come, enough to serve everyone again and again. Besides, soup tastes better as leftovers. Everything is better with time, like distance... (*Her eyes start to moisten. She removes a kerchief from her pocket and dabs her eyes.*) That isn't to say that I didn't love what I had to leave....

NARRATOR

A breeze whirred and hushed. Someone started to whimper. The Old Man wrapped his arms around his wife's shoulders.

OLD MAN

(*To Soldiers.*) I must speak on behalf of my wife and myself, for all of us. You see, we had to flee during The War. (*Belly-Dancer starts to weep. Townspeople console her and one another: Shhhh... shhhh...*)

FIRST SOLDIER

(*Looking around.*) My friends, from where have you come?
(*Among sobs, whispers.* Note: *Numbered Townspeople can be divided among characters, or assigned to audience members. Any number of places can be commemorated, represented by additional Townspeople and/or the Audience.*)

TOWNSPERSON #1

Srebrenica.

TOWNSPERSON #2

Babylon.

TOWNSPERSON #3

Wounded Knee.

TOWNSPERSON #4

Nagasaki.

TOWNSPERSON #5

Robben Island.

TOWNSPERSON #6

Thuan Yen.

TOWNSPERSON #7

Salem.

TOWNSPERSON #8

Dachau.

OLD WOMAN

(*Sighing.*) And so many more. What we carry can't fit in a bag or on a page. We carry griefs and dreams of centuries, so multiplied in our minds that they must fold to fit. Many lie hidden, numbed. We're all exiled in one way or another but haven't found a way to rebuild what is broken.

MIRANDA

(*Coming out of the crowd, pulling her toy pony.*) What we need is a recarved cornerstone, or something of that sort. (*Townspeople turn toward her.*) In my collection, I have many odds and ends, and you can add more, which we can cobble into one great big new stone—as big as the earth!

SECOND SOLDER

Your bag of stones seems bottomless! How have you managed to carry the weight?

MIRANDA

My trusted burro does that. Isn't that right, Dapple? (*She looks to the toy and pats his muzzle with her right hand.*) Apart from him, stones are all I have. All I have left. No one wanted them, so I am their home.

WELL-WOMAN

So! Because of her gift, we won't have to drift!

ALL

This calls for a celebration!

BELLY-DANCER

So be it.

SHAMAN

Let it be.

SECOND SOLDER

Yes—but as for us, we must take leave.

ALL

(*Not in unison.*) Leave?

GRANDMOTHER

You'll not stay long enough to taste the leftovers?

FIRST SOLDER

(*Looking from face to face.*) Thank you for the invitation, and for your generosity. You've been very kind. But we have many miles to travel.

NARRATOR

A breeze caught the brim of his hat and carried it a few feet away. Long hair cascaded down his back, curls that tumbled to the ground, leaving his head bald. He looked like her. Young and old, black and white. The villagers blinked in disbelief until the soldier retrieved the hat and put it back in place.

POSTMAN

Where *exactly* are you going?

BOY

Are you *really* soldiers?

First Solder-who-is-Not-a-Soldier

For the time being, we're like tortoises who carry their homes wherever they go. Our real home—it's hard to describe in relation to here, because it's very far. Suffice to say: Over that horizon and two stars to the right.

Old Man

That sounds very far, indeed. Let us, then, give you some Stone Soup for your journey.

All

(*Like a chorus.*) Yes, yes!

Foster Father

You must take some leftovers—

Young Punk

(*Conciliatory.*) The soup was delicious, after all.

Grandmother

Where you are going, the weather may be cold. You must take three of my blankets.

Painter

And if you want to celebrate anything, here is a bottle of wine!

Preacher

...and two fish...

FARMER

...and a little cart to carry them...

MIRANDA

...and my Pet Rock, Sisyphus...and you may also keep my scarab beetle...

BOY

...and my schnauzer, Pozzo...

THIRD SOLDIER-WHO-IS-NOT-A-SOLDIER

Thank you, thank you! You are too kind.

DOCTOR

...and a life preserver, in case you cross water...

SECOND SOLDIER-WHO-IS-NOT-A-SOLDIER

We'll accept your gifts, if you'll let us share the ledger of stories to spread around the world, so in time, you may find variations of your Stone Soup served back to you. Whether here or there, near or far, someday you may again cross your borders...

OLD WOMAN

How ever can we do that?

FIRST SOLDIER-WHO-IS-NOT-A-SOLDIER

Be patient. You'll know when the time is right.

WELL-WOMAN

I want to go and walk with the foe!

SECOND SOLDIER-WHO-IS-NOT-A-SOLDIER

We're not anyone's foe. We had to appear as soldiers to cross our own borders, and now we must continue our journey. (*Soldier-Who-Was-Not-a-Soldier's eyes well with tears, extending a hand to brush tears from Well-Woman's cheeks. Gesturing to Miranda to join Well-Woman.*) If it's agreeable with my fellow travelers, we'll leave the leftovers in the keeping of this pair. Whenever any of you are in need, please appeal to more-than-one kindness. (*All nod in concurrence. Well-Woman grasps Miranda's small hand.*)

MIRANDA

Wait— (*Steps forward toward Soldiers-who-are-not-Soldiers.*) What if we want to go with you, really and truly?

SECOND SOLDIER-WHO-IS-NOT-A-SOLDIER

(*Surprised, gazes from soldier to soldier, back to Miranda.*) What?

MIRANDA

(*Repeating her question, louder:*) What if we want to go with you? Like the Well-Woman said: to go and walk with the foe?

TOWNSPERSON #1

I do.

TOWNSPERSON #2

Me, too.

TOWNSPERSON #3

And me!

TOWNSPERSON #4

Count me in.

TOWNSPERSON #5

What else do we have to lose?

TOWNSPERSON #6

We're only ghosts, otherwise.

TOWNSPERSON #7

Where? Shall we go?

TOWNSPERSON #8

All of us?

SECOND SOLDIER-WHO-IS-NOT-A-SOLDIER

(*Still surprised.*) We had not considered this possibility...

FIRST SOLDIER-WHO-IS-NOT-A-SOLDIER

How many of you? (*One by one, hands start rising, until all are raised.*)

THIRD SOLDIER-WHO-IS-NOT-A-SOLDIER

(*Gazing at splayed fingers, from face to face.*) This will be a change for us. This will change us.

SECOND SOLDIER-WHO-IS-NOT-A-SOLDIER

So be it.

FIRST SOLDIER-WHO-IS-NOT-A-SOLDIER

Let it be.

OLD WOMAN

Isn't that what Stone Soup is all about? (*Soldiers-who-are-not-Soldiers look to one another, smile and shrug, nodding.*)

MIRANDA

As a Time Capsule, I'll leave behind my collection, since someone may come this way and need stones for soup. (*A few Townspeople bring things to her.*) Anyone else have more to add?

FOSTER FATHER

There's not much to pack, just our cares...

WELL-WOMAN

...having lost all we can bear. (*Goes to console Foster Father.*) Don't despair—

SECOND SOLDIER-WHO-IS-NOT-A-SOLDIER

(*Dispersing containers of soup among Townspeople.*) Our rule-of-the-road is to travel light, taking our needs, giving away wants. Is everyone ready? (*The crowd nods.*)

YOUNG PUNK

What are we waiting for? (*Soldiers-who-are-not Soldiers turn and start walking down steps offstage, into audience. Townspeople follow through aisles, extending hands to invite audience to join the parade; only some follow.*)

SECOND SOLDIER-WHO-IS-NOT-A-SOLDIER

Come whoever wants. Let us go!

MIRANDA

(*Looking around, then off to the horizon.*) Where are we
going again?

FIRST SOLDIER-WHO-IS-NOT-A-SOLDIER

In a word? Home.

MIRANDA

And where is that again?

FIRST SOLDIER-WHO-IS-NOT-A-SOLDIER

(*Looking back to her, then surveying the empty stage.*) Just
be patient. You'll know when we get there. (*Turns to exit.*)

NARRATOR

And so, leaving the cooling cauldron, the townspeople
turned and walked down the stone-littered road, giving soup to
whoever they met along the way, becoming fainter and fainter
in the distance, as they traveled to discover what they already
knew.

Curtain.

II

It is at this point that Boccioni's rupture with Division-ism truly begins....The 1911 painting 'The Street Enters the House' depicts the sitter's circular, all-encompassing experience of the activities on the street by structuring them so they literally interpenetrate the interior space she occupies....When this work was shown in the ex-hibition 'Intima' in Milan in 1911, Margherita Sarfatti wrote, "at La Famiglia Artistica, Boccioni is exhibiting a painting entitled 'At the Balcony' [later retitled 'The Street Enters the House'], in which he means to pres-ent a comprehensive synthesis of all the impressions the woman who is at the center of the painting can experience when looking out her window, including not only the buildings she sees in front of her, but also those she knows to be beside and behind her."

(from Boccioni's Materia)

Famuli tuorum

You sit at the window, beside a lidless jar of museum tags, and watch mummified pedestrians, sharp slanted light, falling snow. The pavement is masked white. Winter outlines ledges. Scuffs of shovels pile slush in gutters between buried cars. Wheels spin, squeaking and grinding, as a car sinks into snowbound ruts. Another car slows beside a woman, whose head tilts toward the opening window, looks at the proffered map, and points down the street.

Here. There.

The car drives away. The stranger heads in another direction in snow, still falling, while you imagine her body, your body – any body – mapped. Not like the city's webbed streets or subway routes, nor color-coded veins and arteries in a diagramed heart, nor opaque splotches on a mind's magnetic map, nor a woodcut corpse from early dissections. Not any of these, but all of them, entwined into something not yet defined. You envision a chart of metamorphoses – modulating, like music – linear yet dimensional, with keys dependent on signatures that progress through expositions, developments and recapitulations, en route to a particular home:

To the home key. Listen, as the woman rounds the corner and leaves the hush of the street, in snow –

A cathedral bell tolls. Through the window, two belfries rise unequally, one unfinished. Its doors are shut, but you've seen them welcome a live menagerie: lions, tigers, bears, bees, snakes, with an elephant wearing an evergreen wreath. From the window, you now see a narrow fire station with a red facade and garage door, open to reveal the cab of a red truck, hook and ladder, reminding you of the middle of one night, one September, when it returned white instead of red, covered not by snow but with ash. That day, bells tolled ceaselessly, after fire and ambulance sirens stopped screaming. And in the days thereafter, when posters veiled the city like snow (as autumn turned to winter), faces of missing loved ones – sought by hair color, height, weight, tattoos, scars, hip replacements, hidden bits of bodies – scattered on shop windows, bus kiosks, lamp posts. Compelled toward them, toward fallen towers, you wandered like everyone, wanting to clear rubble but lacking functional hands, wondering how to collectively keep history from repeating.

The snow continues to fall.

A carillon tolls from your boom box. One bell, then another, quickens on contact, like hammers on anvils. The bells ring in song, then stop. Chanting grows from relative silence, monophonically, then layered, through variations of *Ut queant laxis Resonare fibris Mira gestorum Famuli tuorum Solve polluti Labii reatum, Sancte Joannes....* Shifting and spinning...

Music of the Spheres isn't palpable – if there's truth to the legend. You want to trust something, so question everything: Pythagoras, who bypassed a blacksmith's shop and overheard pling-planging hammers on anvils, calibrating pitches as ratios; Boethius who, before super-strings and quarks, conceived of a

sympathetic vibration among instrumental strings (with the ca-
pability to resonate with, even tune, the universe); Gregory, who
transcribed music from whispers of a dove.

Matins to Compline: one way to mark time.

Blazes of sun; wind; rain; snow –

Winter to spring to summer to –

Morning doves perch on the sill, then fly away. In a besti-
ary, or a Book of Hours. Dominical letters calculate the calendar,
before pages of prayers (framed by thistles, cornflowers, arabesques) conclude with an Office of the Dead. On the margin of
a page *in medias res*, leaves bronze, then fall. A full moon con-
tracts to a crescent, to a squint, then rounds out like an open
eye. Below roosting birds lie beasts, moths, cocoons. More snow
falls. Vines twine around stars and illuminated letters, around
neumatic notations scratched above syllables, indicating ways to
sing the text, presenting a key-that-is-not:

This is Not the Key

Suppose, then, that you wish to commit some
note or neume to memory....you must lo-
cate that note or neume in the beginning of
some melody you know very well. And for
each note to be retained in the memory, you
must have a melody of this sort at your beck
and call beginning on the note in question.
Take this melody, for example: *UT queant laxis
RE-sonare fibris MI-ra gestorum FA-muli tuorum
SOL-ve polluti LA-bii reatum Sancte Joannes.*
    ~ Guido d'Arezzo, "Letter on singing un-
heard songs" (*Epistola de ignoto cantu*, c.1030).
Loose and fragmented translation: "O for thy
spirit... fettered tongues... chasten lips... to
loosen... wonder... be chanted..."

Ut, Re, Mi, Fa, Sol, La, Si – not played by a harpsichord, piano or organ, but sung by an ancient voice that starts to tune something inside you. Animated as breath expires and inspires a body, you want to revive what lies dormant, to reanimate what is dying or merely asleep – or what was there all along, scattered in parts like Echo, whose voice reverberates by answering questions with questions:

Where are you going?

Are you going?

Are you?

(*echoing:*) Dying, or merely asleep? With eyes shut, then opened: *pupils* reemerge (from *pupa* – a Latin diminutive for child, "doll" or "little corpse," a metamorphic insect – pulsing) as you awake from a midsummer night's dream:

La casa entra nella strada: (and vice versa

   revered – a reverie, reverberating)

      Ut queant laxis

         Resonare fibris

            Mira gestorum

               Famuli tuorum

                  Solve polluti

                     Labii reatum

                        Sancte Joannes:

                           diminishing

                           (mirrors, shaped

                        crescents, crescendoing:

                     a Pythagorean comma

                  completes the Circle, dis-

               sonances code the Coda, reverberating from anvils, hammers:

you are beating, you are beating)

resplendent song: a heart –

In the prewar building – rife with doors, leaky faucets,
crumbling walls, clamoring radiators, ringing buzzers, broken
metronome – you sit, cloaked in a moment, a memory of someone
who asked you upon waking, *¿Cómo amaneciste? – How did you
dawn*, she asked, neglecting mention of *sleep.* You think of that
awakening, before and since then, so your mouth fills with words
the weight of stones, impossible to swallow. Outside the window,
dusk sets over honeycombed high-rises, outlined in winter. Man-
tled for warmth, you walk away from the eight-storey window
and start taking leave, dismantling – stone by spoken stone – the
doorframe of your house, your body, which from the beginning
(you were told) was destined to fall, in order to rise.

Ut queant laxis

Galleries don't seem to end – opening into another, way leads to way, into way – she's been here often enough to know she could stay for life and not see everything (could have been yesterday, taped and braced, she was here among dismembered statues but disguised by turtlenecks and gloves, so no one would have noticed, as they read about Apollo chasing Daphne, who branched into a tree, or Daphnis picking a love-apple) navigating galleries, the park, sky, streets that lead to a key in the lock – she anticipates all, after being released from work early, after admitting "I give up" – after taking time (if nothing else) into her hands, to circumambulate the Met before meeting him at:

(Home.)

She recalls his smile, when he'd said, Do you know what I love about you?

She'd said nothing.

He'd said, You have that capacity. To change. You allow the same in me. How would we be here otherwise?

She thought, (I don't know. This is more than a love story: a mystery. Maybe all love stories are mysteries.)

She & he & they & we & you & me – homing:

Toward home!

Not straight away, crow dart-of-an-arrow going home, but a curvaceous, loopy, round-about, verdant waving, weaving (good-bye, hello, good-) course of going home to *Love*, since home is where the heart is, so the saying goes, and she wears it well-fitted all around and inside her, like a snail's shell, able to leave for a hermit to inhabit. She doesn't want anyone to be homeless (even as a state of mind) and thinks while wandering in search of the Ancient Near East – Catal Höyük, Uruk, Anatolia – by way of an arsenical copper ibex stand, cuneiform impressed on clay tablets, ceramic jars, cylinder seals & *kudurru* ("boundary stones"): *What did they bound? Should we cross the threshold?* before "Glimpses of the Silk Road" offer an ivory rhyton carved as a lion-griffin, reassembled from 350 fragments, beside carnelian stamp seals with portraits along the balcony, across from blue & white Ming porcelain flasks, linen-draped tables, baby grand & four stands for a string quartet, since it's almost Friday evening (a performance she can almost hear, Mozart Schubert Vivaldi) – over the ledge, where people cluster like pinwheels among admissions booths, coat checks, the gift shop, information islands, security checks – humming: *La casa entra nella strada: La casa entra nella strada: La casa entra nella strada:*

 Ut queant laxis

  Resonare fibris

   Mira gestorum

Famuli tuorum

Solve polluti

Labii reatum

Sancte Joannes:

(unraveling)

O for thy spirit...

fettered tongues...

chasten lips...

to loosen...

wonder...

be chanted...

In Southeast Asia, she encounters semblances of silence, in a limestone sculpted pagoda enclosing decapitated bodhisattvas across from "Pure Land of Bhaishajyaguru, The Buddha of Healing" (a pigment painting on clay & straw) before a pot-bellied Yaksha and voluptuous Yakshi (male & female nature gods, in stone – that stiffens her thoughts of ephemeral mediums, as she chips away at blocks: to shape all of this, to make it endure, to let go of) bronze metal stupas, inscribed schist reliquaries, a red sandstone Four-Armed Vishnu (missing his conch) & Garuda (with broken wings), copper Shiva as Lord of the Dance & a teakwood meeting hall (whose dome lacks eight large figures, known only from early photographs, of musicians and dancers rising upward toward eight Regents of the Directions, keeping watch) as she goes round, around wider & widening circles, round-about:

Sighing, she picks up pace en route to China, past large

screen paintings with auspicious dragons & waves ("a symbol
of the elemental forces of nature") & fish ("a symbol of unen-
cumbered happiness that is also a rebus for abundance"), past
trailing Japanese *bokuseki* that dance across pages as if alive &
breathing, down a wide marble staircase, whose landing displays a cast iron Head of Buddha, to the ground floor where
visitors swarm and buzz, *See!*

A granite sarcophagus, she sees, then considers en-
tombment within boxes like a nested doll, leaked of thoughts
& heart, bottled and balmed with fractured poetry and incantations, in painted caskets facing a single direction within
walls, ideograms, figures (whose doubled limbs signify movement, following the lion's gaze) – in a hidden room at the end
of a dark tunnel, echoing:

Echoing (empty, empty, empty:)

It is here, where deciphering needs to take place, so far
into the maze. Labyrinthine, the museum is like that, so a
visitor needs a map to find an egress rather than get lost in another gallery, or end up in Ancient Egypt instead of the Exit.

When she sees the tomb empty, she can't move, feeling weighted by stones (broken arms, legs, feet, hands) that
push her inside her thoughts, memories: her escape by grop-
ing in slow motion, like a wind-up toy without a key, raising
her fingers to reach (a key-board, no longer communication,
instead "opening of the mouth" as if to sing) – here, there:
resonances. She keeps believing: temperament is more than
technology, if she listens more closely, she may hear Pythago-

rean commas (slight dissonances) amid Music of the Spheres
(untempered, chromatically) played-by-not-playing, contra-
dictions in terms that grant comprehension, if she listens like
tuners who once distinguished purer intervals – *between the
lines:*

> Go to...
> > Years later...
> > > It was...
> > > > Once upon...
> > > She sighed...
> > Home was...

Retracing routes that brought her here, to trace a new
path, she scatters stones (pebbles or philosopher's) from her
pockets like petals or bread crumbs. And that could be one
way to follow: the story of their coming home – as if larger
forces (aural & planetary motions; the expanding soul & universe) had caused the Fall.

Solve polluti

It was fall when he returned. That fall when Faar returned from The Great War. The first sight the twins saw was his leg. One leg, where there had been two. A brown and green quilt covered him, bulging on his left lap, sunken on his right; a left foot stuck from the bottom, alone. His body slumped in a chair whose wheels left grooves in the orchard's dirt.

Mor pushed him past dusty tracks, oaks, and persimmon trees, toward the porch. The chair rolled sullenly, slowly, then stopped a few feet shy of the gaping girls.

Mor bent over the bandaged head and whispered in his one ear. She placed her palm on his folded hands in his lap and looked expectantly at Eva and Una, who did not move.

Mor's eyes said, *Come and greet Faar.*

The girls stood still. They did not believe the Man in the Chair was their Faar. He had no leg; there was little face to recognize him. They had not seen him for two years, except in the black-and-white photograph that they kissed each night before bed and each morning when they awoke. Days in and out during that interim, Mor had sat by the window, without looking out its unseasonably rain-streaked glass, with her head bent, sewing. She sewed anything sewable in order not to be idle, not to sin. She knitted socks and delivered satchels of them to a building in town, where she also stitched scarlet crosses on white squares, which were joined into Memorial quilts and embroidered with names of faraway soldiers, auctioned to buy more yarn to make more socks.

Though fabrics were scarce, the Memorial quilts were not piecemeal like the Crazy variant. Patterned like occasioned quilts (for births, engagements, weddings, friendships, anniversaries, deaths), they now derived from world wars. The quilt that Mor wrapped around the Man in the Chair was not Memorial nor Crazy. It was Log Cabin style, with muslin rectangles pieced together like the foundation of a house. Mor's quilting companions had called it "Mummy" and "Egyptian" because the rectangles wrapped around a central square—*like tunnels around a secret tomb, on the other side of the world*, Mrs. Gerard had said to Eva and Una, when she described it to them on a visit some weeks ago.

"Come and greet Faar," Mor said aloud now. The girls continued to stare at the Man in the Chair, mummified in the earthy colored rectangles. They wondered if their real Faar was in Egypt, the most foreign place they could conceive. Or if this *was* Faar, then he might be reemerged from a tomb. He responded to "Faar" when Mor called him, but he did not look like the Faar the twins knew. His face held one exposed eye, under which his hollow, sallow cheek bunched into tiny skin folds. The eye looked at them glassily and beaded with tears that rolled down his cheeks, caught and blotted by the shroud that draped his face. He tried to smile, but muscles in his mouth lost their nerve. His pupil resembled one of the apricot stones that littered the yard.

"Come and greet Faar," Mor gulped at the stilted twins. Her pleading gaze gripped them; and their feet crept forward by a will larger than their own. The Man stretched out his shrunken, spotted arms. He tried to say something; but words stuck in his throat. The girls stopped short and shirked at his infirmity. More of his tears came and caught in his cloth.

Not the same Faar, his *datters'* withdrawing expressions said in silence. He saw they did not remember what he had taught them about losses and hidden hearts. They did not think it capable that Faar was so near.

That night, when Mor called the girls to come say goodnight to Faar, they went to his photograph and kissed the small, flat, sepia cheeks of a full face. They did not go near his bedroom.

In the days that followed, the Man in the Chair did not ask to see stars, as the old Faar would have. *So it could not be him*, the sisters concluded. Nor did he talk about the sea or crossing more oceans. At night, he hovered on his bed, shaking and whimpering. Mor lifted him in and out of his chair, wrapping and unwrapping him in his mummy quilt. Her fingers—never idle, never transgressing—found new purpose in bandaging his wounds and sowing the seeds of his farm (apples, pears, apricots, walnuts, persimmons), since two seasons had brought rains that logged the fruits with water, which pulled them to earth and drowned them in sodden ditches. Mor concealed the Man's losses under the quilt and cloth mask, and also strapped on and off his new leg from the Artificial Limb Company, contracted by the State to supply soldiers who had lost parts of themselves.

The Man in the Chair yearned to regain some things but for others desired the luxury of forgetting. There was no cure or prevention against anecdotes that spread in his mind like a disease. No tale could be breathed aloud, he feared, in case it birthed another, more grievous. "Not today," he whispered every time Mor asked.

In the Man's silence, the girls began to concoct tales. The wooden leg became more than a leg, walking around to find its twin, left on the other side of the world, faraway in the Faar-away, in E-g-y-p-t. (How were the twins to know that the bomb had detonated and shrapnel had embedded in F-r-a-n-c-e?) The limb wandered, keeping company with fallen tree branches.

Eva and Una would not touch the artificial limb, not when it was attached to the Man in the Chair nor when it was detached, when he was in bed. Then the girls especially stayed away; when his one eye started to cry and his fragmented body shook; when he pressed his hands to his ear against noise only he could hear and yelled not at them, "Gas, gas!," writhing out of bed, onto the floor, under the bed, fum-

bling and cowering in a corner, legless; his partly faceless face
he covered with quivering hands while Mor ran in the room
and implored, "Lars!," reaching out her trembling hands. The
Man was beyond her grasp, under the bedsprings, under a
spell, shaking and shrieking. Mor slumped back on her heels,
rocked and cried like her ward, and laid down her head to his
level, to be near him. To be.

After a time, his quaking lessened. A moment joined
another moment. He slowly stilled to sleep. His soft breaths.
His. Hers. Both curled on the bare beamed floor.

Those were nights.

As the sun set, it inevitably rose. The Man under the Bed
awoke. Mor unfurled and lifted the tangle of his remaining
limbs into bed. She gave him his memento box to leave open
on his bedside table during the day, though it was stowed in a
hallway chest at night. Inside the tarnished tin-box, a dogtag
lay beside a photograph (of the family before the war, seated
in best frocks and his suit—a copy of the same image the girls
kissed); an empty cartridge; the pen he had used to write letters home; a pocket-sized Bible; and a stack of letters with
crinkled edges, bound with string.

The Man in the Bed did not touch any of the items,
except the last. He opened and closed a particular piece of the
crinkly, scribbled paper, which served as his cache for pressed
petals. The petals were scarlet, fragile, papery like his with-
ered skin, with black flat eyes. He called them *pop-pies*. They
grew everywhere, red, in the Faaraway where he had been.

Their seeds could lie in the ground for years and bloom only when uprooted. Battles had churned up soil across a whole front, and poppies bloomed there as commonly as grass.

The Man in the Bed would touch nothing but the petals.

He was caressing them when Mrs. Gerard came to see Mor. The visitor had organized a bequeathal of fabrics since Mor had not attended a quilting bee in months. "You can make your own design," Mrs. Gerard encouraged Mor, assuming she would make the Crazy kind, given the multiple small scraps in the bag. Mrs. Gerard preferred that non-pattern: the lawless combination of different fabrics, their final union, the fact that a Crazy quilter didn't have to be connected with a particular occasion or pattern, and could add whatever materials she found. *There are enough figurings in our heads, as is,* Mrs. Gerard did not say aloud, thinking of daily tallies of wounded and dead, numbers of battles, gained and lost ground, erroneous estimates of time before the war's end, the date of her nephew's death at Somme, countless funerals before eleven, eleven, eleven, eighteen—too many numbers to want to remember. Colors and textures were safer. Mrs. Gerard removed the pieces, most of which were red or white, among blues, left over from Memorial quilt projects. She also showed Mor thread, needles, and pins in a notion box. "I'll be back in two weeks," the visitor called to the porch as she walked away from Mor, who stood with filled arms, unable to wave.

When her friend disappeared from sight, Mor turned

and walked into the shadowy house, past the playing twins, and down the cool, dark hallway on the creaky bare beamed floor. She continued past the chest that nightly held the memento box, and to the bedroom where Faar quivered beside its openness. Mor dropped the bundle on the bedspread to free her hands, to open the closet door. She turned to retrieve the fabrics.

A single piece had fallen, not on the mummy quilt but in Faar's open palm. Mor tried to remove it. But he held it fast. He unfurled the fingers of his other hand.

Pause.

She placed a second piece of fabric there. He sighed. Mor placed another. *Sigh*. Another. She placed each material in his grasp. One by one. *Sigh by sigh*.

He fingered each piece. The fabrics were soft, feathery, smooth, rippled, ribbed. He lifted them to his cheek, beside the white cloth that bound his senses and blotted his tears; as if there were more to touch than dried petals from crinkled paper. Soft, feathery, smooth, rippled, ribbed. *Sighs*.

Mor decided then: to make these fabrics into a new quilt, of poppies. She would sew a garden of red shades and textures. Although day stole her other energies, night granted her time to work on the project. By candlelight, she stitched. Stitch by stitch, patch by patch; finger pricks dripped drops of blood on seams in silk, satin, crepe, velvet, crinoline; against ruby checkers, paisleys, plaids.

Mor sewed because she thought Faar's heart hid and

could be released. She remembered the old stories—the Giant who Hid his Heart Outside his Body—that she wanted Faar to tell now, to remind the girls and himself. And her. She wanted prayers granted and knew that, if she grew idle, they would not be. If she stopped linking this to that, all would be lost.

She attached fabrics to one another, herself to her activity, irreversibly. Nights spread into days into nights, and days, and more. As the quilt continued to grow, her attention drifted from her *datters*. Her eyes hollowed. The candle burned longer and shortened more quickly than before. When Eva and Una begged for her, Mor told them to keep their own hands busy. "The devil works through idle hands," she repeated and sent them outside to gather fruit, *per-sim-mons*, since those were in season.

Swinging a basket between them, the sisters ran to boughs with pumpkin-orange bulbs. They picked persimmons, one by one, to fill the basket. One of the persimmons burst and coated Eva's hands with pulp. Una laughed and rubbed her hands in the bleeding harvest. And the sisters continued picking, to keep their hands busy. To not be idle. For Mor, for Faar, for Holde, for themselves. For the Giant. For Auriga. For shipwrecked stars. And only after the basket overflowed did they turn back toward home, leaving a flaming trail in the their wake.

Resonare fibris – Solve polluti

A flaming trail: that's what Avra saw. Through the window, in Isabel's backyard, nothing stirred but flaming nasturtiums. Above the flowers, crabapple branches hung plastic birds and chipped mirrors, unmoving. In the window's reflection Avra caught sight of herself, faint and semi-translucent: cropped black hair and slim face.

You.

She.

I.

"I" seemed foreign. For months, she'd looked at herself in the mirror and seen a stranger, too delineated and clear – her twin from another world, almost, in another life, staring from the other side of glass. The window made her appear as she thought of herself: shadowy and haunted.

If only she'd gotten to the fire sooner. She could have saved him, if only...

In Carrie's room, alone, Avra waited for her daughter and mother to return from the farmer's market. Avra imagined Isabel and Carrie walking among outdoor stalls, flanked by a building with a mural of Ferdinand Marcos' head cracked like a piñata, spilling Emelda's shoes. Carrie loved the mural, its bright colors, all the high heels, sandals, and soles tumbling to the ground. She'd recently strewn her room in imitation with her own small shoes.

Noticing her own slip-on shoes, Avra started to walk. As if in search of something, she went to her makeshift room. The first sight she saw was the voice-activated computer. While it hummed awake, she noticed another reflection, faintly: "You," the computer. She had the sense of speaking to it, whatever was inside the box – the Sphinx or Pandora, she'd informally called it – speaking in riddles, *ewe* for *you*, or phrases more garbled or encrypted.

"Who are *you*?" she said, looking at her faint profile in the screen, as it turned from black to blue. The color reminded her of the ocean.

A clock ticked against her hushed breath. *Terra incognita.* The mandala was on the screen, dotted by icons. She opened a new document, positioned her headset microphone, turned on the Sphinx, and said:

" *cap* **Her life began with the see** *correct that* **s-e-a** *period*"

The sentence finished, and the microphone pulsed red. She stayed silent, but words continued to write themselves.

"*Scratch that,*" she said.

The cursor stopped. Webbed marks retreated into blankness. A moment later, new words scurried across the page.

"*Scratch that. Scratch that. Go to sleep.*" She stared at the single sentence. *Her life began with the sea.* "*Wake up,*" she said, "*cap* **Waves rolled outside her window** *comma* **watery raisins** *scratch that* **horizons** *period space space cap* **Her father had disappeared on a voyage into** *spell that* **t-e-r-r-a** *space* **i-n-c-o-g-n-i-t-a** *comma* **where horned no rails** *scratch that spell that* **n-a-r-w-h-a-l-e-s swam under rice** *correct that* **ice** *comma* **where music lulled into frozen flows** *delete that* **flows no no no,**"

Avra stopped narrating and took a breath, which generated "**the.**" The microphone pulsed and wrote "**wind.**" She said, "*Select flows through wind delete that* **flows** *correct that* **f-l-o-e-s** *period space space cap* **She began to dream of loud** *scratch that* **cloud lagoons** *comma* **lead** *scratch that* **belied** *spell that* **b-e-l-l-i-e-d sales** *delete that* **sails** *comma* **end** *scratch that* **and sirens singing into wind** *period space space cap* **The wayfaring hate** *scratch that* **trait had been inherited** *period space space cap* **She decided to wonder** *scratch that* **wander** *period Go to sleep.*" The cursor wrote, **Goes leap.** "Go to sleep," she said, louder. **Goats leap,** it wrote, with the microphone pulsing. Frustrated, she yelled, "Go to sleep!" The microphone pulsed, as if she'd said nothing. Exhaling a long, tense but inaudible breath, she tried to quiet something deep in herself, saying in her steadiest voice, "Go to sleep." The microphone stopped pulsing, turned yellow, and reclined.

Silence settled in the hush.

Waves rolled outside her window, watery horizons, she reread. *Her father had disappeared on a voyage into terra incognita, where horned narwhales swam under ice, where music lulled into frozen floes. She began to dream of cloud lagoons, bellied sails, and sirens singing into wind. The wayfaring trait had been inherited. She decided to wander. Goes leap. Goats leap.*

The clock ticked, slower.

Moment by moment in that rhythm she heard, as if for the first time, what her mind hadn't wrapped itself around, for as long as she could remember: the beat of her heart. It was pulsing. *One, two, one, two.* With amplification from a stethoscope, she'd heard the dual rhythm, diastole and systole, pump and release, a few times. Doubled when she'd been pregnant.

Not like this. This was softer and discernible by imagining the feel of a fist in her chest, *her* fist, clasping and unclasping. Clasp, unclasp. It was becoming her measure against every hum. Beat upon beat, the rhythms aggregated, layering like instruments in a symphony, accompanying something she couldn't yet name. It wasn't even the story that seemed important, so much as the act of listening, of learning to hear.

Beagle whimpered at her feet. She hadn't heard the mutt enter.

"What's wrong? Silly," she added, then remembered Isabel telling her the word's original meaning: "blessed." A glance at the screen confirmed that her voice wasn't being recorded. The mutt rolled around on the floor. *Beagle, not the boat, half the breed. Generically named*, she thought, *my mother spends all day talking Shiva and Mohammed, then names her dog like a cat in an Audrey Hepburn movie*. But Avra was grateful for the dog, almost her best friend now, the only one – apart from the Sphinx – in whom she confided. If Isabel was to be believed, Avra shut everyone else out.

Something creaked upstairs.

"Hello?" Avra called. She listened, grateful for this time alone. It was Saturday. On weekdays after work, the moment Avra entered the house, her mother whirred to the door, summarizing news from the store, where born-again hippies met spiritual bohemians, and travelers learned to distinguish *baraqees* from *abayas*. Avra could almost hear her, describing a young woman journalist traveling to Iran and needing a "raincoat," or a 50-year-old man who'd fallen in love with a Muslim woman and who wondered if he was allowed to weave a prayer rug, or a teenage girl wanting a Saint Anthony medal because she often lost things.

Beagle's tags jingled, as he followed Avra upstairs. In the entry hall, the aquarium hummed, amid bowls for catching leaks. On the wall, a photograph of Isabel was surrounded by index cards with Spanish vocabulary: *abuela* (grandmother), *la boca* and *decir* (mouth; to tell), *las orejas* and *escuchar* (ears; to listen), *los ojos* and *ver* (eyes; to see) – all part of Isabel's plan to teach Carrie Spanish, since she was living in California. As Avra walked into the living room, she noticed a new index card on the *puja* to her *mano*:

tocar = to touch, to play an instrument

The house seemed more and more cluttered with words. It was amusing, in its way. Initially, Avra had worried that the bombardment might confuse Carrie, who was easily adapting (much more than Avra) to their dual life. Avra just needed distraction. Kneeling on the tatami mat, she bent toward the TV remote. A shelf held videos of *The Way of the Buddha. Breakfast at Tiffany's. Living with the Dhammapadha. Infinite Geometry: Islamic Art. Woman of the Year.* She clicked the remote on. The screen flashed colors, a law office, Big Bird, a forest, as she flipped through channels to a map of cloud icons, dotted lines, numbers for temperature, and a forecaster who waved a pointer like a symphony conductor. "...won't stop," he said. "Sports, after this."

"Are you tired of your figure?" asked the Duchess of York.

Avra pressed the channel changer again.

A black background surrounded white letters, *Eternity.*

"...a break today..."

"...fallen, and I can't get..."

"... love me, we're one happy..."

"...one of these things is not like...."

"...Bamenda Highlands of Cameroon, red feathers of..."

The phone rang. Through rooms, Beagle bounded at her heels. Picking up the telephone, her fingers got tangled with the attached index card.

"Hold on!" she yelled, trying to grasp the receiver. "Hello?"

"Avra?"

"Sudan?" she said, recognizing the voice of the manager of *How to Wear a Habit*. He had renamed himself in order to heighten awareness of the devastation in that country. Upon introducing himself to people, they inevitably would remark the name was "unusual" or "beautiful" and ask, "Does it mean something special?" With no Sudanese in his blood and albino dreadlocks, he couldn't sum up his source easily and provided a country's condensed history in place of his own.

"Is Isabel there?"

"No, she and Carrie went to the farmers' market. They should be home soon."

"How goes it?"

"Fine." She wanted to return to the computer but asked, "You?"

"Can't complain. We'd like to see you around here more. This Thursday, a Tibetan bowl ringer is coming. Have you heard her play in the Headlands?"

The reference sounded familiar. Isabel had driven Avra and Carrie into coastal hills pocked by World War II bunkers, overgrown with wild brush. The wind had smelled of licorice and sea-salt. Driving through one of the tunnels, Isabel had mentioned the bowl ringer.

"Yes."

"Some Sundays, they close one tunnel to traffic, and she arranges her bowls to play. You can imagine the echoes and resonance."

"Yeah."

"You should come."

"We'll see. Carrie might not...."

"Bring her, too." The connection crackled, and his voice softened like he was talking to someone else. "Hey," he spoke clearly again, "Gotta go, but have Is call me when she gets home."

"Sure."

"Hope to see you soon, okay?"

"Sure," she said, hanging up and meeting Beagle's eager stare. She thought about Sudan. Isabel had described each of her employees, at length, and said that he was the kind of person who always had time for causes: writing letters of petition to release Prisoners-of-Conscience, accompanying human rights delegations, recycling by exact specifications, participating in environmental campaigns – all while managing the store: *How to Wear a Habit.* How did he do it all? And why work for Isabel? Why did people seem magnetized by her, believing what she advocated without a firm foundation? Or, was Isabel committed to something real? What was real? *But these temporal provisions,* Isabel had written in the Introduction of her first book, *are not ends but rather...."*

What were her exact words? Avra left the kitchen and walked to another index card: *la biblioteca.* She'd only glossed the Introduction of the first volume, not wanting to read when Isabel could see, in case it conveyed interest. But alone, she scanned various editions of the *How to Wear a Habit* series. She slipped the first volume off the shelf and propped it upon the credenza beside an index card (*el corazón* = the heart) among jars of artichoke hearts that still constituted the shrine for Stephen. Flipping open the Introduction, she skimmed the text:

> temporal provisions
>   besides our own habits
>   clothing
>   a wider history of connotations   Latin *habitus*
>
>   condition or character   *habēre:* to have or to hold
> – even to give
>   what is as intangible
>
>   (*ligare*, to link or
>   articulate
>
> temple, monastery, church, synagogue, mosque, and
>
> we come in contact
>   *Given* too   *held* too
> worship may strangle and constrict breath
>
>   the threshold
>   what's inside out
> simultaneously
>   succumb to names and symbols
>
>   the unknown
> behind the   behind the sound
>   breath of our lives
>
> experiences should multiply questions....

Avra closed the book. Her stomach constricted, the way it did when she let herself care. She didn't want to read her mother's words. Hypocrisies – why had her mother abandoned the life she'd been born into, a life Avra barely knew? Why had her father honored the secret of her mother? *I always knew where you were,* Isabel had said, *your father sent updates about you; he was good at keeping my secrets.* Were his letters kept? Would Avra ever see them, ever find an explanation? Was she doing her best for Carrie by remaining in this strange house? Why didn't Carrie ask about Stephen?

Staring at jarred artichokes, she felt her own heart bottled. Her right arm rose to knock over Stephen's shrine, but she caught herself, backed away and almost ran to Carrie's room. The bed lay in shadows. Avra didn't turn on the light and walked to the closet. Hinges squeaked. Inside, her knees brushed against a laundry basket. Kneeling and reaching her right hand toward a pile of odds and ends (ignoring the urn with Stephen's ashes), she found a cigar box.

The container held a plastic compass that Stephen had kept in his desk in the department office, a lens that had been in the car's glove compartment at the time of the fire (and thus was saved), the charred snout of a stuffed Morgan dog that still honked (as it had when Avra was a child, when her father had said the toy was her mother's last gift), a thimble, scraps of paper. She awkwardly unfolded and refolded each sheet.

A few stapled papers were scribbled, scattered details about the Ozarks that she'd researched after Stephen had proposed doing studies and fieldwork at the University of Arkansas. Her handwriting looked foreign. She turned to a flat topographic map with contoured elevation lines and followed a squiggly blue line, south and west where shadings and crosshatches were denser. Her gaze stopped north of Lost Valley, where the Osage had once revered a nearby spring for healing the worst infirmities and extending lives.

The Ozark spring had been reputed as a possible source for the myth of the Fountain of Youth, Avra remembered. She flipped through the stapled papers for that legend; past the map, she found only a photocopy from a *Time-Life* text. At the top of the page was scribbled *American Wilderness Books, 1974, Richard Rhodes,* above underlined sentences:

> The point is that darkness in a cave is like no other darkness anywhere. Outside, even on the blackest nights, with the moon down and the stars obliterated by clouds, the human eye can adapt enough to perceive the dim outlines of the world. But in a cave you literally cannot see your hand before your eyes. There is an alien quality to that darkness, a quality that prickles deep in our bones. It isolates us within our skins, shrinking the world to a sphere measured by the length of our arms, which may be the reason why touch is the most intimate of senses, because it can only communicate news of what has already invaded our vulnerable immediacy, news of what is already at hand.

She remembered the night when she'd agreed to leave Northampton. *What's to lose?* she'd said, unsuspecting. The wire mesh sliding screen, the condensation against her shirt. The night had been humid. Without a breeze. The porch light, the dervish moths, the ratty weave of the outdoor couch cushions, chirruping crickets and cicadas, flickering fireflies, thick humidity, night. She'd sat beside Stephen and folded her legs under her.

If we go, he'd said, as a question.

Yes. It had been her decision.

His fingers grazed under her shirt, around the small of her back, slowly, softly tracing her spine, up around her, pressing; hands following the taut curves and lingering, in the give, the soft grooves. Between ribs and hips. Pressing, compressing. Bone, muscles, tightening, releasing. Flesh. Humid and thick. Night. She remembered opening her eyes as he coaxed her back against the cushions, the ratty weave, the riotous moths, the porch light, flickering, humming, pressed, skin on skin, pulsing inside –

The dry paper moistened in her grasp. She opened her eyes and gazed at the shadowed ceiling. Glow-in-the-dark stars shone in imagined constellations. Even without a lamp, she could see the ceiling webbed with watermarks, delicate lines in cream paint that with time and inattention would spot, flake, and peel. Isabel could decorate a house and store, but didn't know how to care for a structure, to replace leaky pipes, caulk holes, grout tiles, and snake drains. Isabel didn't pay attention to the small repairs that needed to happen behind the scenes to keep a structure strong, like Avra's father had taught her, even as they'd moved from house to house, making each home. He'd taught her to protect herself by attending to one repair at a time, not warning that in one fell swoop, walls could burn or crumble into a pile of stucco, stones, ash.

Something cracked in her, a seal like ice on her heart started to thaw. Her chest, eyes, ears – everything warmed slowly, then pulsed, hot. She bathed in her own heat, listening to her heart beating, suffused by that stippled sound. The house was quiet except for a brief jingle, when Beagle followed her upstairs. In the kitchen, she rifled through drawers to find a box of large matches. In the entry hall, the flaking ceiling reminded her of Isabel, who read patterned cracks like coffee dregs or tea leaves, for fortunes. Signs in every room reminded

Avra that they were living in a house waiting to collapse.

But she wasn't worried about that now, retracing her steps to the altar Isabel had created for Stephen. It took a few tries to spurt a flame. The box dropped. With fire against a page, one corner curled, fringed orange, brown and blackening. In her grasp, phrases smoldered down to words, consuming letters, to singe her skin.

For a second, she thought about setting the entire altar alight. But she moved to the side and let the flame fall into a metal wastebin.

She didn't light another match. The first hadn't been lit to test physical endurance. Saints had walked atop hot coals; *satis* had been consumed in pyres. But Avra wanted to commit smaller acts, in hopes that they might collect into another kind of consummation. Believing that small repairs might help return her to living, as different as living was now, she wanted to burn some small thing she'd loved, not to destroy it – but as the closest thing to an offering as she knew how to make.

Solve polluti

"For those of you who are new," Sister Helena stretched out her black-sleeved arm, "*This* is the beginning." The nun's right fingers touched her forehead, chest, left then right shoulders. "*In nomine patris et filii et spiritu sancti,*" she said, repeating the movement. "Three in One, One in Three: some things Are, that seem unable to Be."

Eva and Una sat to the side of the hot room. Three in One, even as Two. Without Holde, in body at least. Everyone thought they were twins.

The sisters had entered the convent school because their Mor could no longer care, after Faar had shaken to stillness, after his return from The Great War. Mor had stayed by his rotting side, sewn and sewn—undistractable, trance-like— until she slumped into her quilt of fifty-two red squares: a field of poppies that had grown like wild weeds. No one knew about her, or his, deaths until Mrs. Gerard came to visit and found the sisters huddled, mouths smeared with persimmon flesh, shivering under their treasure tree on upturned earth. Mrs. Gerard went inside the farmhouse. The parents were later buried, by the County, in the town cemetery under a single stone, with two names, two births and one death date, estimated, because nobody knew. The sisters were left at the Convent with the quilted garden.

Sister Helena's black cloak rustled and brushed against the desks of Eva and Una—new girls, not yet converted—and dangled the strung beads over their wooden desktops.

"Do you know *this*?" she peered into their faces, emphasizing a word that could have represented anything. The sun glinted off Sister Helena's spectacles, so the girls saw no eyes. Light seared the sides of beads, strung ten-by-ten and joined like a necklace without a clasp, at a cross. The wooden beads sparkled somehow with the kind of shine that attracts nest-building birds.

The sisters appeared hypnotized by the swinging rosaries, so Sister Helena did not wait for their answer. She waddled further down the side row, her black skirt rustling, her arm swinging the necklace toward other girls. "There are many Words," she whispered under her black veil, in colored puffs of sound.

Eva and Una crossed their eyes to see more.

Sun, words, and warmth blurred together.

Sparkling spectacles.

Burnished beads, swirling and swinging.

Purple-red, yellow-orange, blue-green.

"*...B-e-n-e-d-i-c-t-a t-u i-n... W-o-r-d-s*," Sister Helena wrote on the board in billowy chalk script.

B and *R*. *Are* and *Be*. New letters; new vocabulary. Syl-

lable sounds—utterances, meanings unknown—joined together by a roving nun, who returned to her desk, to a box,
and pulled out snake-like strings; who waddled up and down
rows, backlit by sun, handing strands to each girl; whose
mouth kept roving with smooth round letters. *O*, after *J*.

"J-O," she articulated. "Repeat after me, spell in your
notebooks, after *W-o-r-d-s*.

J-O..."

> *j-o*

"...Y-F-U-L..."

> *-y-f-u-l* (filling blankness)

"...space M-Y..."

> *m-y-*

"...S-T-E-R-I-E-S"

> *-s-t-o-r-i-e-s...*

(a mis-heard letter, a variation at work)

joyful my-stories

(in the middle of a page,

under

WORDS)

"*Ave Maria, gratia plena...   ...Benedicta tu in...*
...Sancta Maria, Mater Dei, ora pro...   ... et in hora
mortis nostrae. Amen, Amen," repeated Sister Helena without
taking a breath, bowing her head in quiet animation, her eyes
cast downward.

Slowly, she began trembling, whispering, circumambu-

lating the room in her cavernous cloak. Her necklace of beads
swung, haloed by angling sun. "...One of the oldest forms of
devotion .... Our Lady's joys .... *'kept all these words in her
heart'* .... Remembered, written .... Our Mother's sorrows ...
to share ... with You!" Her arm swept in an arc that included
all the girls. The gesture made her sleeve hang like a broken
wing. She appeared on the verge of rising, swirling her arms
toward the chalkboard. From the ledge, she picked up a chalk
stick and pressed it against slate in cursive, decorative loops
aggregating:

WORDS
joyful mystories
decade

"If you remember one thing," Helena chanted, "Remember this." She pointed at the stack of words. "And this,"
she began writing the first word, *A-v-e*, of two verses to copy
ten times.

G-r-a-t-i-a.

S-a-n-c-t-a.

Other girls—not the twins—bent their heads over their
desks, scrawling, copying. Monk-like. Sister Helena fiddled
with her wimple and the gold band on her ring finger, watching. Clutching beads, she shuffled around the room and saw
ave and *sancta* multiplying under *words, stories, decades.*

Everyone scribbled fervently. Except the pair of new
girls who resembled one another. They sat still, blank faces
with blank pages.

Sister Helena glimpsed their inactivity, their lapped hands, and rustled over to their angular wooden desks, waving two pencils.

"What's wrong?" she gasped at the blank stares. "Just copy," she told them. "Just write what is already written." Sister Helena pointed to the board. The girls continued to stare at blank pages. The nun tried again and grew fluttery, again. "The words are already *there* for you. You don't have to create them." She wrote a verse on one of the thin lines of the paper, where both girls could see. "*W-o-r-d-s*," she spoke each letter, articulately, coaxingly. "Copy what is there," she pointed again at the board. "Before the bell rings."

The twins picked up the pencils and copied, shapes without meaning.

The bell rang.

Twenty girls in gray pleated uniforms and matte-brown shoes gathered their papers, their books, their words, and shuffled from the classroom. The twins, too.

Before long, they began to realize that words offered worlds found in The Source that sat fat on a shelf in the classroom, with blue bindings and gilded leaves. From that, they learned that their cloaked guardians wore *a mode of behavior that becomes involuntary through repetition*. The twins made up meanings for prayers and my-stories, after being taught recitations. They also developed their own incantations, to Holde, to Faar and to Mor: chantable words they had learned before and connected with their yesterdays: *krapp sjø; tun sjø.*

The Reverend Mother chastised, "Do not speak words that are foreign," and separated the girls. Different rooms sheltered their bodies. But each sensed the actions, movements and energies of her double, even distanced. Secret communication in hallways helped. The walls were too holy to be forgiving—whispers echoed around corners and caught attentions of wandering Black Habits that draped disapproval. But the girls learned the nuances of sounds, echoes and repetitions. And of silence. Written verses hid folded, smuggled between notebooks and pinafore pockets. Some ended up buried as offerings to those who had died, while others nestled inside designated vases, hymnals, and cisterns to be found by each other's half.

The sisters found different words, too, to harness their thoughts. *Ubi caritas. Veni Sancte Spiritus. Kyrie eleison. Miserere mei.* At first glance, the language seemed a game of substitutions. *Sancte sjø. Tun eleison.* But increasingly, the twins realized the inequities of words whose syllables split, only to be rediscovered in other words. *Spirit-us. Me-i.* Nothing seemed singular. They tore words apart, to find proof. Of something larger than they could fathom. They tore apart words and discovered the unthinkable: that they, too, could split apart and find meaning without one another, leading them back to some beginning they couldn't explain.

Ut queant laxis – Solve polluti –
Labii reatum – Sancte Joannes

Round & round, she feels as if riding a carousel, but one that stops & starts, so she can get off & on, now that she can climb, mount, hold and move: keeping pace (breathing, absorbing, pondering, while wandering) around hanging scrolls inked with bamboo "In Wind," "In Rain," "In the Four Seasons" & "With Banana in Rain," until she passes through a moon-shaped door, into an open courtyard based on the Garden of the Master of the Fishing Nets, where she stops. Water splashes. Sunlight slants through skylights. No echoes seep from exterior halls. Leaping; lapping:

For the moment, she feels as if the fountain of limestone *feng* ("peaks" made from monoliths set on end) & *jiashan* ("artificial mountains" made from piles of stone), flushed with pink orchids & bamboo – are within her, growing (contrasts of "dark, void, soft, yielding, wet, cool" and "bright, solid, hard, unyielding, dry, hot," *yin & yang*), bubbling & curling her lips into a smile, under a covered walkway (whose open walls "create the illusion of space beyond space…lattice of each window is a different geometric pattern") enclosing & disclosing, so inside & outside fuse (exchanging, bubbling, soothing) as light slips across gray tiles & shadows, evoking Basho's lines: *Even in Kyoto – / hearing the cuckoo's cry – / I long for Kyoto.* Light & time & space invite her inside the half-pavilion across the walkway beside the fountain, orchids & bamboo, to call more words to her mouth, to summon birds like "starlings":

Alight. A-light. A light!

Home!

She replays endings in her mind over & over, of stories that she's beginning to write, a story of living while dying, life's intricate echoes, how many ways she & he could have gone & could go: through doors that are not closed, but opening:

She said –

He said –

You said –

False doors in the museum: she's back in Ancient Egypt, passing unearthed miniature figurines at work in dioramas for the Dead (to provide for their afterlives: carpentry, baking, butchering, brewing, gardening, farming), fragmented inscriptions on wasp-eaten doors, canopic jars (to hold organs, named for the legend of a Greek sailor, Canopus), partial papyri, supplies of linen (with inscriptions sometimes in the corners: "'I' marks were woven on several sheets"), facsimile wall paintings, shards of Dynasties & a roomful of mummies flanked by Artemidora on her bier, dead at age 27, painted & gilded in a red tunic, with snail curls & gold ball earrings (the scarab beetle behind her head acts as "both an image of the

morning sun and the hieroglyph for 'coming into existence'")
– everything echoes, rebirth. Moments condense & confuse
time, as she (the one among statues & foreign tongues, the
one who's going home) observes what she can, glancing *here*
& there, there & then –

She stops. In the middle of the gallery, nowhere particular, randomly rotating, navigating a thread of one story:
"Are, that seem unable to   beginning of   Unraveling:
her mind starts to spin, again: beginning of   the end
blinded   deafening   in dreams   slow motion
her voice appearing   merged into a moan   slightly changed
shape, alighting   in ever-widening   Unraveling: her mind
starts to spin, again: the next subject

                                        taunting

                        textures

          syllables   into the contents

                shuffling   sounds

                forward, back

                                        tangled

          patterns   phrases

                                        shrouded

    Between the lines   another entrance

        rising and ebbing   blurrily-reflected

            becoming manifest

                            rearranged

            decaying image

    no longer   invisible

leaving

you

in front of you

Unraveling: her mind
starts to spin, again, circulating & circling, round & round,
again go you & I & she & he & they & we, seeping out of
marble into paint, oak & gold, dolomite chiseled with faces,
flowering into:

More palmettes & she's on her way again (home, not
straight away, crow dart-of-an-arrow, to *Love*) curvaceously,
by Dendur's tomb with nineteenth-century graffiti chiseled
among ankhs & cartouches, LPOLIT 1819, VIDUA 1820, KI
1872, before a glass-smooth pool filled with pennies that re-
flect ceiling lamps (make a wish), guarded by a red sandstone
crocodile that lacks a tail, under the largest skylight she's ever
seen, which frames tree-plumes like strutting peacocks (eyes
above the obelisk, feathers & fist-clumps of petals, foaming,
ocean-waves) she watches from inside out, but also can't wait
to be outdoors among pedestrians, cross-town blue buses and
bumble-bee cabs (reflecting, refracting through atrium-glass)
she watches them pass, summer autumn winter spring, yes,
it's spring, when the Nile floods Geb under Nut, surrounded
by Nun, in a circular world of dismembered in-

cantations   for those figures who break a-   part
to be re-pieced (O-   siris by Isis, Orphe-   us keeps

singing, playing by

metamorpho-   sing:)

Sancte Joannes

Home was here, where things fell apart. Horace Cragg's thoughts retreated from Una, his dying wife, to sunset-smeared sky, cedar branches traced by snow-edged sea. They lived on an island. Waves rolled along the shore. Through windowpanes, other islands faded in dusk. In his study, Horace stared at Una's loose-leaf notes and disarrayed papers.

Between the lines, he thought, lifting his arm awkwardly to adjust the desklamp. Glow spread over his knuckles, splotched skin, glazed face and hands. Arthritis weighted his joints. His right hip stiffened. The seat of the captain's chair felt like stone.

He hadn't felt this deeply before; hadn't declassified the aches; hadn't wept in the four years of Una's illness. His feelings were filed like research, now disassociating and mixing into her notes, into earlier scenes of her Alzheimer's. When she started to eat a paper napkin at a dinner party and, later, tried to cut herself out of the house with a butcher knife and called him her prisoner – in bed upstairs now, she was palled with odors of decomposed organs, dried blood, talcum. **She** had asked him not to let it go this far, not good for anyone, but he let her last. Unrecognizable. He **wondered**, had he ever recognized her in ages when she'd known herself, when she cast bronze topographies, ever?

Wind brushed the window. His thoughts fell to a frame on his desk. In the photograph, Una stood with their children and her hippie twin, Eva. And Eva's granddaughter (Alice's daughter – Alice, who they'd raised as their own, before she eloped) back when the children were children, living at home and not far away, grown and gone. Now, only Jeanne came every weekend, sometimes with Tobias and their two children, Sandra and Jacob.

In the photograph Una smiled, amid the desk's paraphernalia: typewriter, books, some of her files labeled *Vema, Conrad, Eltanin*. Her career as an artist had been inextricably linked to developments in oceanographic voyages. Since 1947, when a core sediment sample containing ancient shells and modern plankton was collected from the Atlantic Ocean, she'd followed efforts of seafloor **mapping**. The progress had informed her large-scale bronze topographies – from representations of subduction to transform faults to the earth's largest geological feature, the mid-ocean ridge. Most of her pieces were in private collections or installed in plazas of commercial centers. Under highrises, the sculptures of submarine contours sprawled beside financiers eating take-out lunches, crumb-scavenging pigeons, passers-by.

Horace had first visited *Pacific Rim Slice* in downtown Tacoma twenty-five years ago. Toddlers had climbed around the crests and dips of cast trenches and peaks, under approving glances from their mothers who sat on nearby benches. He'd shooed the children, thinking they would rub the ridges smooth like St. Peter's nailless toe in the Vatican. But he'd recently read in one of her notebooks that she'd made *seafloor reproductions on land on a scale where people can walk on* **what is normally hidden** *beneath waves and currents.* That scale – of ambition, of concentration – was a dimension of Una that he loved, he realized he shared: a forthright, if unstated hope to penetrate what was unseen. To apprehend what was unknown. To make it material; meaningful; manageable.

"Horace?"

He tilted his eyes, which caught a slant of light. In the mahogany doorframe stood Nina, Una's former art dealer, retired but still a family friend. Most weekday afternoons, she sat at Una's bedside to let Horace rest. In the doorway, her narrow figure resembled a slim beige hourglass; her lapel glinted with a brooch of curled copper. Gray hair was clipped back from her chiseled face.

"How is she?" he asked.

"The same. You? Where's your coffee?"

"I didn't make any."

Nina raised burgundy fingernails to her chin and stroked her neck. The brooch glinted. "You didn't make any yesterday, either. If your habits were less strict, I wouldn't question the lapse. But you look...did you sleep last night?"

Horace felt picture glass between his fingers, clasping the family photo, before letting it go. He forced a laugh that resembled a cough. "I'm fine. I'll eat something when Jeanne comes."

Nina approached the raised window and pushed it shut. "Aren't you cold?"

"Don't. Please."

"It's freezing."

"Clears my head. I need to finish."

"What?"

"Work."

Her hand lingered on the ledge. "Work? Only on condition that I make you a snack. That's a huge concession for a person who mocks domesticity. If anything, humor me."

"Nina, not now."

She pulled up the window and clicked her nails against the panes. A gust of wind rushed inside. Horace bent his head, reading, and she walked back to the door. "I'm going to leave when Jeanne comes."

He didn't raise his eyes. "Yes."

"Arthur Fenshaw and I are attending a play tonight. Do you remember Arthur?"

Behind her, a sconce lamp diffused shadow; the hallway faded in darkness. Horace's energy drained, as he recalled the artist who'd made multi-media departures from Una's pieces, with representations of Aristotle and DaVinci's theories of **sound transmittance** in water, and of underwater hydrophones that monitored global ocean temperatures, marine mammals, seafloor volcanoes and earthquakes. One piece had incorporated air vents to illustrate how oceans circulate heat around the planet **like ducts circulate heat through a house.** Horace glanced up at Nina's backlit outline, said "Yes," and retreated back into his wife's manuscript.

A shadow fell over the words. Startled, he looked up. Nina hovered beside the desk. Her eyes shimmered.

"You need a rest," she said.

He rubbed his face, looked again; her pupils contracted. The pain in his hip and fatigue in his shoulder increased. He noticed more stiffness in his hands. "I'm fine."

"I worry when you say that."

"Go. To the play. You need time off from...us."

"You and Una are the closest people I have to family. She's like a sister to me. And you're like a brother. I'm worried about you, Horace. I don't know how to say it more bluntly."

"I only want some time to myself." His tone was shriller than he meant. "I didn't think it would go on like this." His voice stilted; muted. The loose-leafs slipped from his hands and scattered the floor. *See what I've done*, he thought.

Nina was already collecting pages, out of order. She patted his hand away gently when he tried to assist, shuffled and laid the miscollated stack on his desk. "If you need anything," she said and squeezed his hand. He looked at her and nodded, without saying a word.

Her steps creaked on the stairs and diminished, until only the sound of wind whistled through the open window. The chill revived him. He shut the open door and leaned, as if **to brace against another entrance**. Under his feet, knotted tassels of

Oriental carpet spread into arabesques and inset diamonds, across pine planks to wainscoted walls, stacked journals and texts, ashwood bookshelves. Worn leather and canvas spines bore names of languages. English. German. French. Russian. Mongolian. Swahili. Tagalog. Australian Aborigine. He reached to touch a volume about Chinook Jargon, then pulled back when the mantel clock chimed more ornamentally than before.

His shirt collar tightened around his neck. His chest constricted. His tongue thickened; it felt as if his heart pulsed in his throat, trying to forge open clamped lips. He had learned vast obscure pronunciations but lacked the ability to say what mattered most, simply, with those closest to him. He thought of his research, after new theories, scholarship, and technology buried his breakthroughs in footnotes. Recently, he'd welcomed requests to write summaries of his past progress – the evolution of phonetic modules and early theories of speech and nonspeech perception – only because he was otherwise forgotten in the field he'd helped to create. Notes on Optophones, frequency-modulation systems, Pattern Playbacks, and other prototypes for reading machines bulged from files, in storage, with boxes of spectrograph films and paints that he had self-manufactured to wet and erase from acetate tape. The relics connected him to the person he had been, the part of himself permanently etched in bylines of esoteric journals, biography paragraphs on dust-jackets of out-of-print textbooks, in university course catalogues. It was proof that he'd amounted to something quantifiable:

Dr. Horace M. Cragg, Ph.D., Department of Psycholinguistics.
Educated at West Point Military Academy and University of Wiscon-
sin, Milwaukee. Lieutenant, Signal Corps, United States Army. Lec-
turer at School of Oriental and African Studies, London, England.
Former Chair and Professor Emeritus at Pacific Crest University,
and Former Editor of JOURNAL OF SPEECH COGNITION, ACOUS-
TIC STORAGE AND OUTPUT HANDBOOK, AND PACIFIC JOURNAL
OF PSYCHOLINGUISTICS.

With the terseness of an obituary, the biographical note
neglected those who would survive him. Phrases summed up
whole chapters of his life. They were classifiable and perma-
nent, while the rest of him seemed to retreat.

A gust of wind drew him to the window. Outside, the sky
spread, dark over fallen snow tinted lavender from the climbing full moon. The brightness of the white diluted the stars, and
its sheen rode along the shoreline on waves. The water crested
and fell, **rising and ebbing** but never rolling the same curls of
foam. His thoughts strayed in the undertow, into recesses of
other seas, dark yet glinting like a metal hook catches shine as
it sinks and waits. Baiting. His mind reeled him back through
ABSTIMMSPRUCHY-YRESTXOHNEXSINN:

shimmering

petrified

bones

echoes

Shuddering, as if from deep marrow. Dusky streaks on the
half-open window confronted him with **blurrily-reflected** dic-

tionaries and wall plaques. *Honor, Achievement* – these and whatever words in black script on certificates, didn't matter. The room
grew cramped and hot; he raised the window. Wind rushed in:

ahàv

love

ayàv

hate

happyo

breath

He stood, almost panting, feeling pulses in his mouth,
peeled paint under his fingertips. His hand grew cold, numb-
ing slightly. His reflection in warped glass appeared furrowed,
gauzy, tangled among pine and cedar boughs and ocean waves.
He seemed like **another person** than that young man he'd once
been, during the War, when he'd learned the Hebrew verbs *ahàv*
and *ayàv*, "to love" and "to hate," differed only by their weight
of breath; and according to Brinkley's Japanese edition, *happyo*
meant "making known to the public," "**becoming manifest**,"
"revealing," "disclosure" and "discovery," without indicating it
was a military term for "messaging" –

The words swirled, **rearranged**, dissolved, and left him
alone with furniture. A table on Singer Sewing Machine treads.
Chessboard of carved ebony rooks, monarchs, pawns. From
a bookcase, more faces stared from a black-and-white photograph: himself as a boy on the lap of his mother, before she died
in the influenza epidemic in Stillwater, Minnesota. She'd never
smiled in his memory, as hard and long as he'd tried to reimag-

ine her. Too many years ago.

Creaking, below the bookshelf, a globe turned slowly from the wind (*or something more?*, he wondered, impossibly) on a waist-high wooden stand – "your world," his father had said of the gift that had cost his savings, when Horace left for West Point. That globe had turned outdated continents and oceans on its brass axis, then and now, until Horace planted his finger to stop the revolutions, on Honshu, like a belated prophesy, then traced meridians to the nearest latitude, to a seam in the paper surface that Una had peeled like an orange, when he'd first met her.

The clock chimed. Wind whistled through the open window. Pages on his desk rustled. Horace gathered them, spooled paper and carbon into the typewriter carriage. He shuffled hastily through reproduced reconnaissance images, photogrammetry manuals, bathymetric and acoustical maps. Adjusting his spectacles, rubbing his right shoulder, he read his wife's handwritten words *of knowledge that distinguished...* His fingers grazed the space bar; as he typed, keys clicked: *C-o-n-s-i-d-e-r t-h-e t-e-x-t t-h-a-t s-h-e k-e-p-t b-y h-e-r b-e-d-s-i-d-e, a w-o-r-n h-a-r-d-b-a-c-k o-f P-h-y-s-i-c-a-l G-e-o-g-r-a-p-h-y o-f t-h-e S-e-a. I-n i-t-s t-i-m-e, M-a-t-t-h-e-w M-a-u-r-y w-a-s a s-o-l-i-c-i-t-o-r o-f s-o-r-t-s....*

Hesitation; rereading. *Solicitor of....*

Una – she. Her **decaying image** blurred his pace. *Consider the text*, past the paper – his gaze strayed beyond the Olivetti to a letterhead tucked in the stampbox, addressed to her, *to com-*

memorate increasing interest in oceanography and the science, his-
tory, and art of related disciplines.... commissioning a series of auto-
biographical and biographical articles.... Given your contributions....
honored if you agree to our request.... two pieces, one of an oceanog-
rapher.... and you.... The rest of the letter folded under the crease.

You. He'd thought to replace the "hers" and "shes" that he
was writing with "I" and "me" – "the text beside *my* bedside."
But as he attempted to write *her* autobiographical article, everything he felt dissolved **between the lines**. Where to start. The
paper crinkled as he pulled it from the carriage, crumpled. He'd
never rendered a life and knew that to chart one chronologi-
cally, with a definite beginning, meant giving it an end. A linear
progression **no longer** seemed the right direction. Round and
round, like revolutions of the globe, he wished the center would
roll and each could return: Una. Jeanne, Graham, Rachel, even
Alice – as distant as he was from himself, as Una was, maybe
as they always had been from each other. The people he should
have known best, he knew least. Horace wanted each of them
to come around again, as he had first known them. He wanted
to be given another chance.

Slowly, prompted by the text or something more, his
mind retrieved words from blankness – phrases that she'd told
him, if he could remember. He thumbed forward a few pages in
her manuscript to a transcription of *knowledge it afforded, the*
remote corners of the earth, he skimmed: *closer*

two oceans

air and water

visible, the other **invisible**　　　*underfoot, overhead*

　　　　　meeting – battle, dwelling

　witness rage utmost　　　　　　　　*fury*

　　　　　　　sea, earth,　　　*air;*

　　　entering　　　　　　　　　　　　*both*

　　　　　　unstable

　　　　　　　　equilibrium....

"Dad?"

He looked up, unfocused. A young woman stood in the doorway. At her knees, a boy with plastic red glasses clutched a lunchbox. Jacob, his grandson. His daughter Jeanne spoke again.

"You didn't answer the phone." She wrapped her arm around Jacob's back and nudged him into the room. He dropped his hands to his sides, still clasping the box handle. The contents rattled. Jeanne undid its clasp and emptied pine blocks on the hardwood floor. The boy sank to the shapes.

"Why didn't you answer? It's freezing in here." She sounded tired. At his desk she grasped the phone's receiver and looked at the base. A knob was switched to the right beside *Ringer Off*. "I got you a new phone for more frequent communication. Then you choose to learn *this* technology, when you ignore all others." She paused and shifted her weight. "When was the last time you wound the grandfather clock?" She went over and pulled the pendulum.

"It's been chiming."

She looked at the stopped time, then at him with creased

brows, and fidgeted with the clock-hands and chains, until tick-
ing resumed. "If Nina hadn't answered mom's old phone line, I
would've worried the whole ferry ride. You live isolated enough
on this island."

The clock chimed and pealed seven tones. Horace looked
down at his desk like a guilty schoolboy. Jeanne walked to
the window and shut it, cutting the whistle, and said, "Nina's
leaving."

"She left."

"No, she didn't. She stayed because she's worried about
you. Dad?"

Horace followed the shadows under his daughter's eyes,
hazel. Like her mother's. He searched for something to ask
about. "How are **you**?"

"Been better."

Horace took a deep breath. "How's Tobias?"

She glanced at the clock again and moaned. "I've got to
call him. He's not coming tonight because Sandra has a slumber
party. They'll come tomorrow morning. If he can leave the lab."
She glanced at her son.

Horace clenched his brow. "Did his grant get funded?"

"Yes," she snapped.

Horace swallowed his next question.

She glanced again at Jacob, then back at her father's gaze,
and sighed. She walked to Jacob and tried to lift him; he pulled
away and reached for more blocks. "Can you watch him while
I'm downstairs?"

Horace nodded, but Jeanne wasn't looking. He thought of
Tobias, how alike he and his son-in-law were, although they'd
never been close; how he wanted to say to him now, *Don't miss
what's right **in front of you***.

"Dad, did you hear –" her pitch rose.

Their eyes met. He nodded again.

She left without closing the door. Her footsteps creaked
on the stairs. Murmurs reminded him of Nina's glinting brooch,
of dark circles under Jeanne's eyes.

Jacob knocked blocks to the floor. He grinned as they
scattered and clapped his hands, which Horace thought Jacob
couldn't hear. Or could he? Did he hear inside himself? Like
geophysicists mapped submarine contours by echoes, could
sound vibrations be perceived through fluids inside his body,
as tremor or echo?

The clock chimed. Quarter past the hour. Jacob continued to play, as Horace stuffed papers and carbons in a drawer of
his desk. Warped glass reflected his actions and the interior of
the study: antique globe, foreign dictionaries, gooseneck lamp,
grandson. Stippled in the window, the old man unclasped his
wife's pages, sank to the captain's chair, closed his eyes and
bent forward, as if listening to the last beats of someone else's
heart.

Solve polluti

This was the **beginning of the end**. Eva's heart pulsed, as she remembered Sister Helena's words. Ages ago. *Some things Are that seem unable to Be.* She clenched pages wrapped in butcher paper and twine. Reflective windows glinted, too bright. The sky **blinded**, as she bound along streets in a faded gold dress, shielding her eyes, peering down at cracked sidewalks. Honking horns and shouts. Light taunted her to gaze up again at molten windows. The sky creased with a soaring cross, shrinking and tilting – a plane, quartering a reddened sun, momentarily – until the orb again glowed full.

Et antiquum documentum Novo cedat ritui.

Supplementum Sensuum defectui.

Tantum Ergo.

Quiet descended, **deafening**. *Ergo, Sensuum, Novo.* Her hands burned. In scorching heat, she stopped, dizzy against a building. A few blocks later, she snuck through pews of a cool church, lit by stained light. Catching breaths. She clenched her pages tighter, returned outside and walked at the sun's mercy, instead of retracing steps to Una's apartment to rest.

Three in One, even as Two: separated on different coasts of the country. Days before, Eva had ridden a train, reversing the journey that Faar once had made. She'd brought all her savings from work – as a clerk for a department store, secretary to an editor, proofreader's aide, court reporter – all to get her story out of her hands.

In the cramped dark room, Eva barely saw Una, but reacquainted with her sister through her studio. Canvased with paintings, sculptures and clippings, the room held a window with a fire escape for a balcony. It blazed with heat. Sticky humidity left Eva tossing at night, restless and jittery by day, especially in mornings, as she brought pages from publisher to publisher, who turned her out to fevered streets.

With little to eat, Eva remembered how to relish rations, to yearn for sleep so bread and wine might come to her **in dreams**. Deprivation refined her hunger, as she descended underground and back to the surface on trains, loosing herself among strangers. Inside rolling clouds, thunder growled and screeched. Lightning spurred storms, when she stayed outside, tilting back her head to swallow rain, waiting to be quenched. **Listening**. The sky cleared, again and again, day after day, until she felt something growing inside her—

The city seemed to tilt, again and again.

Leaving Una's balcony, Eva wandered warping streets and avenues, dodging shards of sky. She sought cover by pilgrimage, starting at an old Fort. Cloistered corridors resonated with echoes. Under paling dusk, Eva tried to recall what had happened on the other side of the country: with the old newspaperman. She gazed across the river at shriveled cliffs, trying to remember *M.E.*

Water coursed around the island, sweeping to the Harbor. The next day, at the top of the Empire, she watched more of the sky fall, piece by piece, viewed with a bird's eye. Ant-sized pedestrians scurried and dodged in **slow motion**. Heat seeped until she felt chilled. Gold slivers littered the street, like ice calved from glaciers, reflecting and refracting the sun, melting. She started to lose her hands. Then, her knees. Pearly eyes and shriveled ears riddled the street. Una was nowhere to be found. Everything, gone, but a skeleton of sky, snuffed in smoke. As for Eva, **her voice** seemed to be disappearing, too.

The river beckoned. Beside whispering waves, alone but not, she sensed something physically changing. Past a squat red lighthouse, she followed a path into brush. A kite bobbed. Hinged wings danced, then disappeared, as the trail meandered. The kite reemerged, caught a draft, whipped up and tossed.

The air buzzed. Flattening and cooling. Muddy lulls. Humidity dissolved into shivering. A girl emerged from the brush, holding the kite's reel, tilting her face in slow motion – **appearing** like Una and Eva, **merged**, years ago. Holde? The air hummed **into a moan**. Freezing, Eva listened and looked through absent ears and eyes, trying to remember, scanning the river and opposite shore: for Una. Faar. Mor. Glimmers splintered the current, angling and undulating, as the river flowed fast. The kite flew into what-was-left-of-the-sky.

The girl disappeared. The moan diminished to a hum, beneath faint gushing water. Air stiffened again with humidity, thick and hot. A cry rose, out of view behind trees. Birds twittered, as Eva's senses separated. Her hand was wet. She looked down to find a dog licking her palm.

The dog sauntered away.

Afternoon passed.

As she returned to the heart of the city, mirages consumed pavement. There, a pond. Persimmons. Red petals. Cranes flying above plains. Mountains and forests swelled through slivers, budding between skyscrapers. *Salve, Salve.* Branches of blossoms fluttered into birds. Scattering W-o-r-d-s. Horns honked while the crowd rushed Eva off the curb, into the street.

Standing near the sidewalk, she gazed through trees and laced light, to windows glinting. Holde, Faar and Mor – she hadn't thought of them in years. She wanted to dig deep into earth to find a ghost-blue bone.

A bird dove from the sky, out of sight. Her thoughts spun filaments, weaving into wings. A **slightly changed shape, alighting** to move blood around her body. Circulating. She stood in the street, then wandered **in ever-widening** circles, until a policeman pulled her back to the curb.

Before departing the next day, one last trek led her through labyrinthine streets past pedestrians, hitched horses, too-pale statues. She still clutched pages to her chest, and buildings still tilted. But the sky had reemerged blue with pink-fringed clouds. At the edge of the East River, a walkway crossed The Bridge. In the middle, unbinding twine, she dangled over the ledge. With a single fling, pages fluttered toward churning water, a dispatched flock, like carrier pigeons whose **wings (not free, but entrusted)** couriered messages to someone waiting back home.

Resonare fibris – Ut queant laxis

Home. Here. *For now,* Avra thinks, gazing down at churning seawater. *Not going backward, but forward.* Waves toss. A gust of wind buoys her jacket like a cape. Her cheeks sting, chapped. Sunbeams pierce fog above the Golden Gate.

Carrie runs ahead to the platform deck.

The spreading ocean reminds her of Una's topographic sculptures. Two weeks prior, Avra had visited *Pacific Rim Slice* and some of the smaller works when she drove with Isabel and Carrie to Washington, for her great-aunt's funeral. Neither Avra nor Isabel had seen Una in years, but her funeral had brought an unexpected reconciliation. Forced in a car for a few days, Isabel had started to share her life's story and filled gaps where Avra's memory butted up against imagination. Listening more to each other, mother and daughter had been trying to start a new chapter – less based on who they were in the past, more on who they had become.

"I don't see anything," yells Carrie, walking back up the stairs. "It must be high tide."

Looking out at the coastal opening, Avra's thoughts stray to Point Reyes, faint in the distance: 100 square-miles butting against the mainland on a different tectonic plate, moving north an inch a year, like a slow-sailing ship. That kind of change – unnoticeable to the naked eye – gives her hope.

"Come on," Carrie pulls her arm, "Let's go to class." Turning up the road, Carrie clutches her sketchpad and sprints past cypresses and eucalyptus, toward a palatial white building. Avra follows, focusing on her daughter's path. Neoclassical columns flank the museum's courtyard, where glass pinnacles split the pavement like iceberg tips. Avra pauses to look at an original cast of *The Thinker*, but Carrie circles back and tugs her arm, repeating, "We'll be late."

The prior weekend, Isabel had taken Carrie to the first of three drawing classes: a birthday gift. But earlier in the week, she'd insisted that her daughter and granddaughter make their own outing, offering her car and helping Avra rig a mitt to grip the steering wheel.

Navigating galleries, Carrie leads Avra without asking directions, all the way to the classroom door, and barely waves goodbye. Watching through glass, Avra marvels at the ease with which her daughter mingles.

"You can pick her up in the Rodin Gallery in an hour," says a voice, "near the main entrance – the gallery with the organ." Avra turns to an outstretched hand and tinted tortoiseshell eyeglasses, framed by a black bob. "I'm Dee, one of the teachers. Your daughter must be Carrie? I'm a friend of Isabel's." Avra introduces herself, and Dee rattles off themes of current exhibits. "And around the corner, there's a new one about Music and Art, small but worth a visit."

Avra dawdles in the hallway for a moment, then wanders toward the exhibit. Making a few wrong turns, she enters a small gallery with vibrant canvases in gilded frames. A placard quotes:

MUSIC BEGINS WHERE WORDS END.

Barely does she finish reading when a couple approaches. A petite woman with the decorum of a docent accompanies a gaunt man in a tailored gray suit. Avra follows their gazes to a veritable explosion of color, and gasps. They're observing the cover art, framed, of the novel that the bookseller had given her months before: *The Street Enters the House*. Not the cover, but the actual painting, hangs before her very eyes.

"This is one of the most provocative works for me," the woman says in a gravelly voice. "A *strada entra nella casa*, a Futurist painting by Umberto Boccioni, 1911. Notice the bursting hues." Her small, sleeved arm gestures like a wing. Light glints off her pearl necklace. "I've seen alternate translations, including *The Street Enters the House, Street Noises Invade the House,* and *The Noise of the Street Enters the House*. What intrigues me in relation to this exhibit is the emphasis on *noise....*"

The man stoops and tilts his head toward the painting, as if listening to "a single picture plane," while Avra catches bytes: "without multi-media... noise... sonically conflated with visual... Noise... colors, numbers, letters... blurred senses..." Avra eavesdrops as the woman points to other canvases, *The City Rises... rrrrreddest that shouuuuuuut and greeeeeeeeeeeens that screeeeeeeam... dynamic arabesque in Music, colored notes on a canvas... typographical harmony...*

Rrrrrrred. Greeeeeeeeeeeen.

Upsidedown, rising. My-stories—
       krapp sjø   *tun sjø*
             disembodied
      aháv   *ayáv –*
la casa   *hidden*

                                    entra   nella
          strada   *turning*
                      kaleidoscopic
              el cuento
                  desaparecido
                      twisting:

The man squints in his suit. He seems aloof yet timid, as if his constitution relies on stinky cheeses and vintage wines. Stooping closer to the woman and closer still to the canvas, his face contorts and relaxes, intermittently with his mouth slightly agape, as if inhaling emissions from the painting. Scrutinizing textures and edges, he stands close enough to kiss the canvas, almost neglecting his companion's words:

"...appropriated, dissociated, and re-contextualized to evoke a broader sense of human experiences, by using the sensibility of sound. Or more specifically, music. Take this piece by Vermeer over here," the docent glides toward another frame. Avra follows the *Music Lesson*. A black-and-white checkered floor leads to an upright virginal, where a maid stands with her back turned, poised to play. A gentleman watches from the side. A mirror above the keyboard reflects her slightly upturned face and part of the artist's easel.

The docent turns toward her companion. Her voice drops to a whisper. Avra moves to hear, but they walk away.

Keeping distance, Avra strolls around the gallery. Colors and shapes flare from frames, as clatters and twangs meld with voices and footsteps. Mumbles mix with captions, shimmering

lutes and flauted trills, illuminating *Young Girls at the Piano* beside red, blue & yellow-gridded *Broadway Boogie-Woogie*, swirling faster as circuits connect the black-gloved *Singer at a Café
Concert* with *Compositions & Improvisations*, arrangements in gray
major & keys of black, shifting through reds & greens & blues in
The Wedding, smooth & staccato bamboo keys on gourds (*mbiras*)
beside a headless Makonde drum with feet & navel & breasts (*li-
kuti*), lilting violins & strung harps & curvaceous cellos (*Le violon
d'Ingres*). Winging whistles surge from Saint Cecilia's portative
organ, wreathed in clouds (Calliope, Melpomene, Polyhymnia,
Euterpe & myriad muses, inside music, inside a museum: remembered) in a collage, piecing together Music of the Spheres
from pentagonal & hexagonal designs in Islamic tiles, a Roman
mosaic of Orpheus, arabesques in oils; *are those stones weeping?*
– listening & circling, energized again by a circle of hands in
The Klinger Quartet, near a glass case with a trio, she smiles at a
smiling terracotta *Drummer/Singing Storyteller* unearthed near
thousands of sculpted soldiers in the Sichuan Province; marble
Cycladic *Seated Figure with Harp*; more hands on a harp, like Klee,
but from a tomb's fragment in the Valley of the Kings – then,
Le temps menaçant appears by the *Reclining Woman with Organist*,
rippling rose-hued *Marguerite Gachet*, & a copy of *Schubert at the
Piano* (since the original burned during the second World War)
beside Cubist guitars, *The Ambassadors* with vanitas, *Attributes of
Music, A Humument* ("sing through the hushed ear" "the sound
in my life enlarges my prison"), illuminated vellum with neumatic notation, staves & saxes, *trompe l'œils* & oils on canvas,

Self-portrait: Hesitating between the Arts of Music and Painting... Music... Mosaic... Muses... *Me excuse...*

"Excuse me," repeats the docent.

Avra turns to face the odd couple. The symphony in her head crashes like cymbals. The gallery echoes strangely.

The woman stretches out her arm. "This is yours. We saw it slip off your finger." Her hand opens to reveal a gold band.

"My ring." Avra gasps, lifting her empty left hand, then her right. Her mind thrums with diminishing sounds. Her remaining three fingers are thin, ghostly pale, tinged blue. "It's been loose. I didn't feel it slip off. Thank you. I... you... I...," she stammers. "I have to get it re-sized."

She takes the band and smiles. The odd couple stares abstractly, almost through her, before turning to the next painting, resuming their talk. Avra watches with slight unease, then relief, as she fiddles the band on her finger. She's never taken off the ring except for the operation. Now, it sits gaping, so she removes it again, pulling apart Velcro in her coin purse to slip it inside with spare change and Chinese cookie fortunes. Seeing her partial hand, she feels exposed. Memories swell as her palms open. The room expands as paintings prompt her to hear & feel & lure her from her shell that calcified after the fire. Warming to a flush, her heart races. Her skin tingles. In anticipation, alone now, she relaxes.

Twangs from the Tinguely sculpture intermingle with hushed footfalls and murmurings. Out of the corner of her eye, Avra notices the docent's mouth move. She steps within earshot back beside the painting where the pair started. The woman looks as if she doesn't know how to smile, amid "vibrations... lametta, chevrons, chirascuro... A *strada entra nella casa*... moves, runs, turns... never stationary... appears and disappears... incessantly... galloping... four legs, twenty, triangular... angled light, splintering... tricks of nature... *States of Mind: Those Who Stay, Those Who Go, The Farewells*..." *Leaving home, going home, leaving*... "interior and exterior, open and closed, public and private spheres, confinement and release..."

The docent looks directly at Avra. And smiles. It's the kind of smile out of place with her decorum in the gallery. "I'd like to finish here," she says to the man and to Avra, "with *The Noise of the Street Enters the House*. Although I don't care much for the Futurism Movement, I do appreciate its *movement*; and I almost hear something when I look at this painting. It makes me wonder what might be created by extension, using today's milieu, as we understand more and more how movement itself – our ability to move – the movements that make us and that we make, restructure our consciousness..."

Her voice trails off, as a piano begins to play. Avra looks around the room, sees no instrument yet recognizes the notes progressing slowly through cadences, pulsing and pointillistically accelerating into waves.

"You're listening to 1955," says the woman. "Glenn Gould, interpreting Bach's last *Goldberg Variation*, written in 1742. Gould wrote a decade after this recording: 'forty years ago the listener had the option of flicking a switch inscribed "on" and "off"… Today, the variety of controls made available to him requires analytical judgment.'" She pauses. "Let the Jacques Loussier Trio take it from here."

Avra gazes from painting to painting, then closes her eyes to envision the materializing music. Piano notes parade tightly; rhythms start pushing a more syncopated beat, adding percussion, improvising in ways that she hasn't imagined but which seem natural to this variation on a Variation. She feels her body wanting to move; her head bobs slightly. "The Noise of the Street has entered the House," the woman says and turns to take the man's arm, without another glance at Avra.

Leaving the gallery, their bodies blur and shink from view.

Avra rubs her eyes.

Suddenly, she remembers Carrie and asks a bystander the time. Exiting the gallery, she walks the same direction as the elusive couple. Variations follow, fading into hushed footfalls and whispers.

Following a cave-like stairwell, Avra arrives at the main level and finds her way to the Rodin Gallery. Lit by a grand skylight, the entrance faces a pipe organ. Museum-goers and sculptures on podiums dot the hardwood floor. The room muffles with echoes. Toward the front, Carrie sits cross-legged with the drawing pad in her lap. Sketching energetically, she seems oblivious to the crowd and to Avra, who approaches quietly, focusing on Carrie's subject: two marble hands pressed palm to palm, large enough to hold a human head. The travertine branches with beige veins, fading into yellowed rock, into knuckles, joints, fingers. Two hands appear as one, carved from the same stone.

Before she can take another step, Carrie sees her and clutches the sketchpad to her chest. "I'm done," she says. Avra doesn't ask to see her daughter's drawing. There will be time for that, she feels certain. Like there will be time, if she stays open to the possibility, to make amends with her mother and her past, sifting through variations of her grandmother's life to understand her own.

They leave the gallery and make their way out of the museum. Back in the car, Avra steers the car nervously to residential streets. Carrie points to gulls circling above Seal Rock, wooden windmills at the edge of the Park, gray-green ocean. Wisps of white streak the blue sky. Beyond the Zoo, they arrive at Fort Funston, where Avra parks. Carrie carries a large paper lunch sack. In her arm, Avra cradles a smaller box: Stephen's ashes.

Near the sandy cliff, bright hanggliders flock. A few, already airborn, snake through the sky. Twisting and swooping, their handlebars glint. Midday sun backlights their illuminated wings.

A wooden observation deck provides seats for bystanders. Dogs scurry around children and couples. Avra and Carrie point at the colored gliders and talk above shushing tides, far below.

"Let's go chase waves," Carrie says.

"You lead the way," says Avra, already standing, grasping the container of ashes. They descend rope-ladder steps against a gentle slope, past sea fig and flowering iceplant, erosion nets and beachcombers with wet dogs. It takes almost fifteen minutes to reach the water. Low tide has stranded seaweed, shells, hermit crabs, and driftwood on damp sand. Barnacle-encrusted pilings of a washed-out pier disappear and reemerge, as waves rise and retreat.

Carrie drops the paper lunchsack and coos about unbroken sanddollars. She starts collecting. Avra sits on dry ground and opens the container of ashes.

The breeze shifts. A few grains swirl upward.

She pours some ashes into her left palm. Capping the container, she holds the handful as best she can.

Carrie taps her arm. "You're it!" She jumps backward and runs away. As Avra follows, ashes slip through her clenched fingers. Wisps of clouds, pelicans, and hanggliders circle above their chase. The ocean foams. Mother and daughter trip around nipping waves and a washed-out sandcastle. Avra tries to keep her partial fist clasped. Finally, her fingers open. Ashes fly above the surf. She watches them go. Carrie watches, too.

"I can do that!" Carrie yells, picking up a handful of sand and letting it blow in the breeze. "Try to catch me," she says, starting to run again.

Avra doesn't move, to run or scatter more ashes. Wanting to save remaining ashes for other days, other outings for Carrie to recall, she imagines a trail of breadcrumbs they can follow back here and into their future. She opens both hands again, asymmetrically holding her palms to the wind, letting herself go.

The tides spit foam, fizzle and churn, as more waves gather and rush the shore. Sand mashes between her toes as she calls Carrie back to the blanket. They eat, then lie back to watch hanggliders circle. New colors, zigzagging patterns. Distant ones spark like fireflies. Sun bleaches the sky's blue. Avra closes her eyes and feels her heart pound. Saline breaths. A small moan: Carrie falls asleep. Avra feels her own eyelids descend, hears the waves hush, fainter and fainter. Slowly, a pitch clarifies into a cadence, as she too falls toward sleep, rippling and rushing: *Home. Home. I'm going home....*

Ut queant laxis

$\mathbb{H}$ome! Home! You're going home! Not straight away, crow dart-of-an-arrow going home, but a curvaceous, loopy, round-about, colorful waving (good-bye, hello, good) course of going home – to *Love* – not by plane, train, coach or car, but by foot through labyrinthine halls and echoing galleries, vibrating as marble statues lack legs, hands, noses (breathing); floor-to-ceiling canvases, blue nudes & strung guitars (listening), head-dressed gazelles with locked horns, beaded earflaps, iron mudfish in pendant masks (murmuring). Like a whorled conch, ringing:

Home!

You're going home!

By following arrows. Arabesques. Next text. Next. *Look!* (the gallery, captions, your memory:) Where did it begin, & with whom? (Homing: Honing: Home:) And more: galleries don't seem to end – one opens another, way leads to way, into way – you've been here often enough to know you could stay for life and not see everything (could have been yesterday, taped and braced, you were) navigating galleries, the park, sky, streets that lead to a key in the lock –

you anticipate all, after being released from work early, after admitting "I give up" – after taking time (if nothing else) into your hands, to circumambulate the Met before meeting me at:

Home through the American Wing, flying past grandfather clocks, wing chairs, baseball cards, Madame X's black V-neck, Wright's arithmetical room & Tiffany glass lampshades before Arms and Armor. European Sculpture and Decorative Arts. Medieval Art. Almost crowing, dart-of-an-arrow (yet still loopy, round-about: would you wish for this straight?), you weave, verdant waving (good-bye, hello, good-) course of going home to *Love* through tessellated fountains, fired tiles & calligraphed niches & woven carpets – all tangled together like vines in a jungle – as you (the one who's going home) unravel & ravel anew. You don't have time to circumambulate all galleries today & must leave something to return to: another wing, another room, another skylight (like the one above Rodin's marble chained prisoners, whose massive hands – you're always noticing hands, opposable thumbs, driving forces behind human evolution & the creation of art, communication, technology, social organization – remind you of the French sculptor's unfinished hands, arms, heads, legs & torsos, heaped in his studio & nicknamed "brushwood"), stopping only to glance out the window at leafage flitting (humming) among plumed petals, ocean foam, fluttering masts & hooked anchors (homing) on the other side of glass, in the park, light splintering inside clouds, as you think of:

Home!

You're going home!

Not straight away, but drifting & shifting shapes, birds & butterflies & bees, amid maples & oaks (drifting & shifting, who seem to be whispering *shhhhhh* from another season, exposed, *shhhhhhh*ivering, like autumn, remembering autumn, that Fall); as sounds echo, reflecting & refracting the spectrum (violet, indigo, blue, green, yellow, orange, red: hue of the expanding universe), as you retrace routes that brought you here, following stones (pebbles or philosopher's) like petals or bread crumbs, to trace a new path. And that could be one way to follow: the story of our coming home – as if larger forces (aural & planetary motions; the expanding soul & universe) had caused the Fall.

Fall, falling, falling in love....

It began like everything else, indirectly. Curling at edges, unexpectedly reflecting, refracting the chance meeting in the arch, you & me, beginning without ending – the Circle of Fifths offering another beginning: *It's alright*, I said & you echoed, *Alright*, I haven't told anyone here in this city, where I moved to be a stranger. I don't want to explain. Tell me more about you, I'd rather hear.

I said, Why?

You said, Why what?

I said, Why do you trust me?

You said, I don't know. I just do.

I said, Thank you. For your trust.

You said, And yours. I didn't mean to –

I asked.

You said, I should go.

I said, I want to see you again.

You almost resisted but, instead of leaving, asked, Are you still a musician?

I said, During the day, I manage. And you?

You said, I'm a teacher, a student. A writer. Of sorts.

I said, There are crossovers. What are you writing?

You said, *The House Enters the Street.*

I said, What's that?

You said, Stories within stories, between the lines.

(The light slanted. The crescent moon grew full.)

You told me later: about replaying endings, over & over, after we were no longer me & you – instead, *we* – how many ways we could have gone, through doors that aren't closed, but opening:

False doors in the museum: here we are again (lost & found) behind & ahead, you remember ankhs & cartouches & a pool (make a wish) as you bypass unearthed figurines, dioramas for the Dead, canopic jars, partial papyri, fragmented inscriptions, unlearning to learn: always there's heading to & from. Not one particular place, but orbiting two (three, four, five) at once, how we laugh about mutual coincidences, tomorrow & today, apart but together, with thoughts of & for the other (in our own miniature painting, the horizon line rises) yesterday, connecting & bisecting, pulling apart & repiecing

(meyou, youme) again & again & again, slants of light converge
& illuminate paths coincidentally crossed & re-crossed (where
we met: in the arch, by the fountain, on the beach, again & again
& again, re-pressed keys & hammers & anvils & strings: music
plays between lines): *here* or *there*, *now* or *then*: reunion could
have been anywhere or might never have happened at all. At once
you remember (a dream? *Look!*) – past & future echo in galleries,
sweeping through rooms like underwater waves, water & light,
past gallery guards, skeins of choir screens, *wunderkammern*,
mirrors, inlaid armoires, teardrop chandeliers, brass astrolabes
& compasses & timepieces (watch-hands: going!), sloughable
as luminescence (to cast off every season) as you sprint earlier
& later, closer & farther, to & from:

Home! Delight! Anticipation! Dart-of-an-arrow
like a crow, you're getting closer (if you can, sprout wings
to fly) past pedestrians in jeans & suits & sweats & strollers,
as much as you love Rembrant, Vermeer, Blake (all about
light, *burning bright*) you'll bypass them to revisit another
day (always leaving something – Kahlo's cracked mirrors,
Dali's melting clocks, Warhol's Campbell's cans, Grecian
Urns & Exquisite Corpses – to come back & see & hear)
children asleep or giggling at guides who murmur mysteries
about Rapa Nui phalli, gathering in the Great Hall (en route
to Arts of Africa, Oceania, & the Americas) among audio
guides, sketchpads & notepads & hearing aides & wheelchairs
& maps & coat checks & information islands – homing &
humming. A tune, recognizable, on the tip of your tongue

beneath the balcony, where it plays, makes you pause to listen while pocketing a metal M (tags collect in a jar at home: pink Ms, purple Ms, green Ms, yellow Ms, millennial Met) & walk out of the museum empty-handed, without looking over your shoulder, keeping the tune in your head, intervals unraveling, heading past tinged bronze windows, streaming with sunset, marbleizing into golden eyes, blinking at a wide sky:

Opening! Getting closer! You're going – straight as you can (among sparrows, pigeon-holing) speed-walkers, roller-bladers, bikers, venders, dog-walkers: rambling through the Ramble at a sprint. It's spring, early in the season when buds verge on blooms, pink & yellow & blue edging a palatial turret on a hill, glowing in silhouette, petals bursting upon sky among crabapple & strawberry fields, hopscotch squares & green kites with trailing tails, whirling, lilting like the rising cadence of a song (lulling) sky to ground, carpets unfurling from fallen blossoms. Heat palpates inside buds, whiffs of breeze, feathers of birds, bees & butterflies curl & unfurl (birds, bees, buds) not autumn-loss nor sunset, but: dawn-pink, dawn-violet, dawn-golden. Petaled apparitions of faces bow from boughs, brightly, from branches where sunlit chorales lift, from birds & a carousel, camouflaged by limbs like clasped fists that hold petals, fluttering fingerlings, unfurling tidal foam (crests & crashes & hushes) dispersing flocks of sea-birds. Alight! A-light!

A light hawk inks the sun, sea-clouds, peacock plumes, flying higher across the sky, circling then descending over a

boarded green theater toward a rock of carapaces, clawing &
glinting in a mossmurky pond, landing on a turtleback and
cocking a lidless eye, before realighting –

Sun slips behind a cloud. Tonal shift. *Grâve*. In that
moment: spring falls back to winter behind ice, freezing what
came before & will again. Leaves, fallen. Time slows. Glistening
icicles, lace traceries, crystal sills: in that season (everything has
a season), you retreated inside, slowed your pace in the too-long
winter, cold and confining, what kept you climbing walls (of
your mind, of your voice) with your useless hands in your pre-
war apartment, where a radiator pissed steam and leaked tears
on the hardwood floor, like a steel-heat accordion – plinking,
sighing, hammering – under the sill of a window that framed
a frozen world. It was a long winter, but then came melting:
crocuses, popping through snow like butterflies from cream
cocoons; buds, like mist among foaming clouds & shimmering
sun; you, unwrapping bandages and braces, molting & reaching
out to unlock windows, opening the bolted door of the pre-war
apartment to navigate halls, leave your house & enter the street.

Sun seeps through the cloud, shining. Tonal shift.
Allegro. The reservoir glistens with emeralds & diamonds
(you feel rich, blossoming around the lake & on water,
golden crabapples & ornamental cherries) dispersing a gaggle
of goslings, who ripple wakes, glide across rings & waddle
ashore into flaming brush. Along the running path, smudging
footprints: you sprint home past trees, geese, jewel-strewn
reservoir under canopied petals, through the park back to

the pre-war apartment where the radiator is off, windows are open so air moves freely inside & outside into the kitchen, living room, study, dining room, bedroom (there're all one, in a studio), where I'm headed at this exact moment, 5:00 p.m. (done with work for the weekend) so we'll meet & make dinner, dicing & sizzling orchestration – Von Bingen, Bach, Chopin, Villa Lobos, Pärt, Tan Dun – they're all there and more, in the pre-war apartment, where music sings from the stereo & seeps out windows, under cracks in the door, through walls, into music that keeps playing. For us, it is not a silent world.

You said, What's this about?

I said, It's a love story.

You said, Truth is stranger than fiction.

I said, What do you believe?

You said, Everything. Nothing.

I said, Us?

Back then, we were in the park, under a crescent moon. It was autumn. You looked up at bare limbs of trees, down to your empty hands.

You said, Do you know what it means not to be able to carry simple things: books, jars, your body? If this worsens again, I may have trouble opening every door.

I said, Let me –

You said, I can take care of myself.

I said, That's not what this is about.

You said, I'm making a new home.

I said, Do you know what I love about you?

You said nothing.

I said, You have that capacity: to change. You allow the same in me. I said, How would we be here otherwise?

You later answered, This is more than a love story: a mystery. Maybe all love stories are mysteries. Back then, you said, Truth *is* strange.

I changed the subject, Tell me more about what you write.

You paused, then said, Lost things. Things I've lost. Not always directly.

I said, What have you found?

You said, Everything. Nothing is everything.

You are, I said. I feel like I've come home.

Love, you think, *Look!* At the sky, at sea-clouds, ocean waves, ebbing and rising, white numbers in red circles, paved stairs leading down, down, down (*listen:* rumbling) turnstiles and newspapers, rats & rattling, light at the end of the tunnel, approaching. Lights, bells, voices! The loudspeaker announces, "We're being held by...." *Poetry in Motion*:

"Living" –

A red salamander
　　so cold and so
　　　　easy to catch, dreamily
　　　　　　moves his delicate feet
　　　　　　　　and long tail. I hold
　　　　　　　　　　my hand open for him to go.
　　　　　　　　　　　　Each minute the last minute.

"...3 a.m."

A single light
  Where someone
    Was sick or
      Perhaps reading
        As I drove past
          At seventy
            Not thinking
              This poem
                Is for whoever
                  Had the light on.

"The Suitor"

....turning all at once
  like a school full of fish.
    Suddenly I understand that I am happy.
      For months this feeling
        has been coming closer....

Commingling with commuters, lights & loudspeakers, you recall the afternoon today, your life, all time, dawns & dusks, shifting earth & sky, paperbacks & paperbags, bebop from the duo who enters the subway from the end of the car, "Spare a dime, anything you have," tinkling cups, *10¢ a minute long-distance*, Subtalk *<<Add wings? <<Ban automobiles? <<Convince customers to exit at the rear....yes, that's it!*, SOMETIMES YOU HAVE TO GO BACKWARD IN ORDER TO MOVE FORWARD, "Stand clear of the closing doors," opening, closing, opening, closing, gathering momentum, speeding through the tunnel, slowing heeeeeere, heeere, her:

Who (you)? Where (here)? Why (hear) –

Home! You've arrived, at the nearest station stop!
Sliding doors open, & you bound up the stairs, two at a
time, glance at your watch ("Next stop...") can't come
soon enough (home, home, home) through rows of light-
twined trees (breathing) out the quad through black gates &
stoplights & sirens under an overpass (down, down, down)
at a moderate slope past *The Last Word, Ye Olde Appletree*
near the intersection (listening), where you turn & start
skipping under the purple-tinged sky, bronze clouds &
honeycombed windows which appear at twilight (echoing,
home) on the verge of daylight savings, turning night into
day & day into night, shifting, shadowing & illuminating – a
light in our window, I'm home! Hear: Home, ehom, meho,
omeh, home, ehom, meho, ooooooooooooommmeh. You
rush inside the U-shaped courtyard past planted urns to a
switchboard, don't stop to find keys, buzzing in signature
rhythm. Call & response: a bell answers back, & you push
open the door (can do that now, open a door by yourself –
a good spell, you're having) coming in from twilight, into
the warmth & low light of the pre-war foyer of the pre-war
building, where your entrance (lapping & leaping, the front
door smacking shut) echoes against the mosaic floor & metal
mailboxes (goodbye, hello, good-) leaping up stairs, as your
soles skid against tesserae tiles, to reach the second floor &
turn down the mosaic hallway, where you hear the click of
my bolt, unlocking:

Coda

Thus they went on living in a reality that was slipping away, momentarily captured by words, but which would escape irremediably when they forgot the values of the written letters.

~ Gabriel García Marquez,
One Hundred Years of Solitude

Famuli tuorum

Sift your fingers through double-braced barrels of kernels of corn. You have no trouble grasping, at this moment in time. Gather handfuls of kernels to fill the basin in your arms. At the village pump, swizzle the parched seeds. Keep water flowing. Pump and release, pump and release: the action requires repetition, muscles solidified by labor, strength you have not previously needed. After cleaning the kernels, shuttle the basin to a lean-to with a fire kindled before dawn. Twigs poke from a hollowed-out stone that will blister your touch, if you don't take care. Beside the hot rock, there's a tarnished grinder; grit grainy paste through the shredding sieve. The paste should hesitate, then curl before falling onto a rolling slab. With a pestle passed down through generations, urge the pulp flat, flatter. Gather the cohesion into a ball to shape between your palms. Turn it forward and forward, rotate and pat, again. Flat. Your circle is thin, but not supermarket thin, palm-sized sustenance that you place raw and imperfect (since you are learning) on the scorching stone to sizzle. Pockets of air rise as it heats, freckles and browns. Remove it to add to the growing pile of steaming disks wrapped in a cloth, warm.

You eat the tortillas with her, a grandmother. You talk of

lost children and wait. As boiled milk cools, your tongue burns. Too hot: wait, so ground cinnamon won't stick to your lips. The milk came from a goat across the lane, offered after it bleated and kicked and a knowing hand cradled its neck, to calm. The hand was not yours because you are a foreigner; you do not know how to assuage a goat, or the meaning of calm. You watch, hungry for knowledge not learned in books, imagining the wise fingers on your slender neck. Greedy eyes, she calls you in soft laughs, as she senses you want to be generous but are learning.

You forget that sunrise is a habit because you have no blinds on your windows. Instead of glass, wooden sockets frame a vegetable world. Banana trees, coffee plants, and palms grow lush among deheaded cornstalks, hollowed houses, stone-littered roads. In afternoons, thunder grumbles over the valley. Silence defines sound because it is evasive; there is always the undermurmur of cicadas and the river.

At night, too. There is always the undermurmer of cicadas; the river. Behind the buzz, breezes, bombs. Under murmur. Guns. Fire. Don't breathe, or scream. This happens again, as before: through wooden shutters, skeins of sunlight sketch hammocks as colored cobwebs, pinned among sleeping bats, hidden wings. Droppings scatter a doorway, lit by dusk, an uninhabited yard: hollowed stone oven, an awning, rusted drainpipes, scuttling chickens, hole in the ground. Under your hammock, moonlight seeps around shifting bodies. Creaking beams. Snoring. Rustling. Screeching. Dark arcs slip out the door, flights soft as whispers. The sky cracks, stars. Falling on the ground, you crawl to a cracked wall to see: stars in the street, dancing; the neighboring house a flame.

Say-ee-say-a-day...not a word.

Cicada. Say, *cigarra* –

See *guerra* –

Sí, sí, sí –

Through the valley, the river rims a dusty road and twists from your surrogate community, *Las Vueltas* ("the turns," you learn the meaning), to villages beyond the verdant ridge, pocked hills, mountains, camps, bordering there:

A route of repatriation.

Here, she comes behind the lean-to through the dirt yard. It's night. A candlelight's ringed glow catches her shadow as she raises her wrinkled hand to speak. To you. She trusts you with words: how the soldiers came and took her pregnant daughter, opened her on a rock, and made birth a double funeral. She thinks you will protect stories like you protect your own life, no, longer. You learn the fecundity of stories, how one gives birth to another, and cradle her words as she taught you to nurture tortillas, to rotate them, again and again. She grasps your unblemished fingers before disappearing into darkness.

*   *   *

Repeat after me:

re   pi   ta
re-pi-ta
repita, por favor =
please repeat

Me di ga
Me lo diga
Dígamelo

diga = Ud. form of root-changing irregular verb *decir*
decir = to tell
me = pronoun replaces direct object, *yo*
lo = pronoun replaces indirect object, masculine antecedent
un, el cuento = a, the story
escuchar = to listen

es   cu   che
es-cu-che
escuche

lis   ten
lis-ten
listen

Ab-u-e-la, cuén-te-me-lo.

el   cuen   to
el   cuen-to
elcuento

the   sto   ry
the   sto-ry
thestory

– *Mi hija, escuches. El cuento. Me apena decirtelo.*

I do not want to bring you pain. Do not tell.

– *No comprendes. Los cuentos son las vidas. Apuntan por la verdad.*

The truth? I don't yet understand *la verdad* or *la vida.*

la vida = life

presente!

presente!

presente!

I'm listening. By this candle in the yard, I see you. I hear you.

– *Mis niños.*

Your children?

– *Están desaparecidos.*

> *desaparecer* = to disappear, vanish; (~de vista)
> to drop out of sight
> *desaparecido* = missing; extinct; dead

Your four sons and daughters.

– *No.*

I misheard, or was something lost in translation?

– *Es verdad que tengo cuatro niños. No he visto a tres, pero vi
a mi hija. Hijita mia...*

> The letter *j* + *vowel*, like the combinations *ge* and
> *gi*, have no English equivalent; the Spanish is
> pronounced at the back of the throat, forcing the
> air through a narrow opening.

You saw one of your daughters? Where?

– *¿Qué veas?*

> The letter **u** (pronounced *oo*, as in tune) in *que* or
> *qui* is always silent.

What do I see?

– *Miras la milpa.*

Cornfields.

– *Y los plátanos, cafetales y campos de yuca...*

Yucca, yesterday. The roots are difficult to harvest, tangling in soil near the stream.

– *El rio...*

The river?

– *Viene de las montañas y de la lluvia....*

You showed me where it comes from the mountains. To bathe, there and in the rain. It rains heavily as if the sky were weeping.

– *Miras la aguja y el hilo.*

The needle and thread, on your lap?

– *Los hilos son como las personas. Si una puntada se desenreda, la cadena se desenreda.*

> *puntada* = stitch
> *cadena* = chain; bond, link; series, sequence
> *desenredar* = unravel

– *A causa de la guerra.*

una, la guerra = a war, the war

causa, efecto = cause, effect

efectos personales = personal effects (a patch

of clothing, a thread, a tooth, photograph

in a pocket, a finger, a handwritten prayer)

– *Mi esposo murió.*

Your husband, lo *siento*, lo *siento*. Many lives lost.

– *La guerra. Más años que tú. Más años que yo.*

cuántos años tiene = how old are you? (*formal*)

cuántos años = how many years?

cuántos = how much, what amount?

a) *los desaparecidos*

b) *los muertos (75,000)*

c) *la guerra*

ch) *Yo, Tu, Ud, Uds, Nosotros, Vosotros*

(me; you *informal*; you, he or she *formal*;

them or you-all *formal*; us or we-all,

informal)

– *Miras el pueblo.*

In this town, I live with you. You've been like a mother to me.

madre mia!

madre mia!

madre mia!

– *Las madres y los padres no están aquí. Viven en las monta-*
ñas. Luchan por los niños del futuro.

I've been through mountains with you. Past the river through fields and forests, to camps hidden among trees. Those who hide are willing to give their lives for children, those who are and aren't born.

– *Soy una abuela.*

You're a grandmother.

– *¿Y tú? Sábes la expresión para 'vida nueva'?*

*¿Cómo se dice....*the expression for 'new life'?

– *'Nacimiento.'*

'Birth'?

– *Sí, 'dar luz.'*

'To give light'?

– *Literalmente y en sentido figurado.*

Literally and figuratively.

– *Como la sangre.*

Like blood.

– *La sangre riega las semillas de la liberación. Riega las rosas
de la U.C.A.*

>   *regar* = to water (a plant, a garden)
>   *las semillas* = seeds
>   *U.C.A.* = Central American University at San Salvador

I've seen the roses blooming in a circle on the graves. You called
them a miracle. They've not stopped blooming, even in winter.

– *Que no se te olvide.*

I won't forget. You teach me to remember.

– *No olvidamos. Juntas. Yo y tú.*
(We will not forget. Me and you.)

*   *   *

re   pi   ta
re-pi-ta
repita, por favor =
please repeat

diga = tell
cuento = story; tale
cuenta = counting; reckoning

*   *   *

How did you sleep, Grandmother?

– No comprendo esta expresión.

When you see a person in the morning, how do you inquire
after her night's slumber? *¿Cómo se pregunta por la calidad del
sueño?*

> *preguntar* = a, the question
> *calidad* = quality
> *sueño* = sleep, dream

*– Entiendo. No tenemos esta expresión. Preguntamos, ¿Cómo
amaneciste?*

A different verb than 'to sleep'. *Amanecer,* 'to dawn'?

– Sí. ¿Cómo amaneciste?

How did *I* dawn?

– Esta es mi pregunta para ti.
(This is my question to you.)

*   *   *

It's still night. Under murmurs. *Cigarras.* Cicadas. *El rio.*
The river. The generator is broken. But you've learned to listen,
to see by the moon and by bugs that light like stars. Fireflies.
Their glitz bursts so expectedly at nightfall, stars seem less common and are distilled by nearer-orbiting, new constellations. You
catch the fireflies in an empty Coke-bottle glass. The bugs fill

the hollow with glow – you do not consider the grasp as trap-
ping. It becomes your flashlight. You trip giddily over reflective
cobblestones with your live lantern and laugh like a drunk trying
to suppress loss of control. The stupor implodes. Your shriek escapes before you catch it, freer than the bugs that flit slower and
slower in their transparent cage.

Ceci

n'est

pas

la fin:

Acknowledgements

"Gratitude" shares etymological roots with "grace" – as in, *to be honored by your presence*. Thanks to you, dear reader, for picking up these pages and to those readers who helped bring this book into being. To the editors at Starcherone Books, particularly Carra Stratton and Florine Melnyk, who believed in this novel and encouraged its publication, I am ever grateful. With his committed colleagues, Ted Pelton has been a wonder of a publisher; it has been a pleasure and privilege to partake in his vision for fiction. Many thanks to Claudia Esslinger for enlivening Umberto Boccioni's already pulsing painting for the cover, and to Rebecca Maslen Sapolsky for working her graphic magic on the alphabetic dimensions of the book. The two images reproduced for this novel include: Umberto Boccioni, *The Street Enters the House* (*La strada entra nella casa*), 1911, Oil on canvas, Sprengel Museum Hannover; and Guidonian hand, from a liturgical miscellany, Italian, late 15th century, UPenn Ms. Codex 1248, Rare Book & Manuscript Library, University of Pennsylvania. Thanks to Peter Pürer and Nancy M. Shawcross for their assistance with permissions to use these images.

The House Enters the Street is a work of fiction; any resemblance to actual situations or people, living or dead, is coincidental. I am indebted to many writers, artists, musicians, and others who have inspired me over the years. In lieu of length, thanks to those who have worked across the range of literature and beyond, interrelating language with other evolving arts; who have vitally and vibrantly melded content with form; who have invited new ways to question, perceive, and inhabit the world through words.

Many sources inspired this novel, and I am grateful for their contributions. The novel's epigraph comes from Marco Polo's *The Travels of Marco Polo: The Complete Yule-Cordier Edition* (reprinted by Dover Publications, 1993), 4. The dual section epigraphs come from captions to paintings by Umberto Boccioni exhibited in *Boccioni's Materia*, mounted at the Solomon R. Guggenheim Museum in New York (February 6-May 9, 2004), organized by curators Laura Mattioli Rossi and Vivien Greene. The epigraph for the novel's Coda comes from Gabriel García Márquez's *One Hundred Years of Solitude*, trans. Gregory Rabassa (New York: HarperCollins, 2003), 47. The excerpted libretto comes from the aria by Giacomo Puccini in *La*

Bohème, "Mi chiamano Mimì." The quotation about medieval solmization, attributed to Guido d'Arezzo, is discussed and translated in Piero Weiss and Richard Taruskin's *Music in the Western World: A History in Documents* (New York: Schirmer Books, 1984), 44. The line from William Blake's poem "To God" can be found in John Sampson's edition, *The Poetical Works of William Blake* (Oxford: Clarendon Press, 1905), 235. Arturo Francamano's fictional restaurant, "The Holy Palate," both derives and departs from F.T. Marinetti's experiment toward a Futuristic dining experience and cookbook. For the dramatic collection of that same name written by Nova Francamano, her epigraph comes from a poem by Robert Penn Warren titled "Tell Me a Story," collected in *New and Selected Poems 1923-1985* (New York: Random House, 1985), 230. "The Girl Without Hands" is included in *The Complete Fairy Tales of the Brothers Grimm* (Hertfordshire: Wordsworth Editions Ltd, 1997), 164-166. Dragon NaturallySpeaking inspired the novel's voice-recognition software called "The Sphinx" (loosely representing an early incarnation of the technology, but not the actual software's current and more accurate capabilities). The voice-recognition training passage comes from Lewis Carroll's *Alice's Adventures in Wonderland, and Through the Looking-Glass* (New York: Macmillan, 1897), 32, 37. The passage about darkness in a cave comes from Richard Rhodes's *The Ozarks* (New York: Time-Life Books, 1974), 47. Quoted fragments of text by Matthew Maury were first published in 1855 in *The Physical Geography of the Sea*. Goethe said, "Music begins where words end," and Tom Phillips's *Music in Art* (New York: Prestel, 1997) aided the related fictional exhibit in this novel. The poems framed as "Poetry in Motion" in the New York Subway include Denise Levertov's "Living," Donald Justice's "Poem to be read at 3 a.m.", and Jane Kenyon's "The Suitor." Among other sources, this novel is deeply indebted to the Metropolitan Museum of Art.

Excerpts from *The House Enters the Street* first appeared as stories in literary journals under the following titles: "Where Are You Going?" in *Alaska Quarterly Review*, "The

Mummy Quilt" in *Ascent*, "Appearing" in *Eleven Eleven*, and "Las Vueltas" in *The Iowa Review*. Special thanks to the editors and staff of these journals, particularly Ronald Spatz, W. Scott Olsen, Hugh Behm-Steinberg, and David Hamilton. If Rikki Ducornet had not chosen this manuscript as runner-up for the AWP Award Series in the Novel in 2005, it likely would have disappeared in a box of abandoned projects. Many thanks to her and to others who encouraged me not to fully unravel this modulating manuscript. Binnie Kirshenbaum has been a touchstone over the years, as has Marly Swick. Beyond fellowship support for my graduate studies at Columbia University and the University of Missouri, I also am grateful to an array of teachers and classmates, not to mention wonderful students. Thanks to Mary Gordon, Ben Marcus, and Carole Maso for their kind words about the book, and to individuals who read sections of this manuscript at various points: David Plante, Karolis Zukauskas, Kathryn Harrison, Heidi Julevits, Nathan Oates, Amy Wilkinson, Trudy Lewis, Nickole Brown, among others who shared support, including Kate Dunn and Amy Greene. The Writers' Colony at Dairy Hollow provided a month-long residency at a critical time. The earliest seeds of this novel were watered by the dedicated teaching of Jonis Agee and Alice LaPlante. Before I could fathom being a writer, John McPhee taught me to map narrative through his elegant sense of structure. Fritz Norstad, Marie Ernster, Susan Ackerman, John Murphy, my parents, brother, family and friends first taught me to care for stories that connect, inside and outside, with a wider world. Abundant thanks to each of them.

Naming seems to neglect those who are not named. People not thanked here also have had profound effects on my ability to create this novel, and my gratitude is unbounded to each of you. Last but never least: my deepest love and gratitude to Ethan. He can never be thanked enough. Wherever we go, he is my home.

About the Author

Gretchen E. Henderson is the author of the novel, *Galerie de Difformité* (winner of the Madeleine P. Plonsker Prize). Her other books include a work of nonfiction, *On Marvellous Things Heard*, and a poetry chapbook, *Wreckage: By Land & By Sea*. Gretchen is a Mellon Postdoctoral Fellow at MIT.

Colophon

The fonts used in this book are Georgia for *Famuli tuorum*, Baramond for *Ut queant laxis*, Berylium for *Solve polluti*, Gentium for *Resonare fibris*, Museo Sans for *Labii reatum*, Liberation Serif for *Mira gestorum*, and Chapparal Pro for *Sancte Joannes*.

Also Available from Starcherone Books

E. R. Baxter, *Niagara Digressions*

Kenneth Bernard, *The Man in the Stretcher: previously uncollected stories*

Donald Breckenridge, *You Are Here*

Blake Butler and Lily Hoang, eds., *30 Under 30: An Anthology of Innovative Fiction by Younger Authors*

Joshua Cohen, *A Heaven of Others*

Peter Conners, ed., *PP/FF: An Anthology*

Jeffrey DeShell, *Peter: An (A)Historical Romance*

Nicolette deCsipkay, *Black Umbrella Stories*, illustrated by Francesca deCsipkay

Sarah Falkner, *Animal Sanctuary*

Raymond Federman, *My Body in Nine Parts*, with photographs by Steve Murez

Raymond Federman, *Shhh: The Story of a Childhood*

Raymond Federman, *The Voice in the Closet*

Raymond Federman and George Chambers, *The Twilight of the Bums*, with cartoon accompaniment by T. Motley

Sara Greenslit, *The Blue of Her Body*

Johannes Göransson, *Dear Ra: A Story in Flinches*

Joshua Harmon, *Quinnehtukqut*

Harold Jaffe, *Beyond the Techno-Cave: A Guerrilla Writer's Guide to Post-Millennial Culture*

Stacey Levine, *The Girl with Brown Fur: stories & tales*

Janet Mitchell, *The Creepy Girl and other stories*

Alissa Nutting, *Unclean Jobs for Women and Girls*

Aimee Parkison, *Woman with Dark Horses: Stories*

Ted Pelton, *Endorsed by Jack Chapeau 2 an even greater extent*

Thaddeus Rutkowski, *Haywire*

Leslie Scalapino, *Floats Horse-Floats or Horse-Flows*

Nina Shope, *Hangings: Three Novellas*

Starcherone Books, Inc., exists to stimulate public interest in works of innovative prose fiction and nurture an understanding of the art of fiction writing by publishing, disseminating, and affording the public opportunities to hear readings of innovative works. In addition to encouraging the development of authors and their audiences, Starcherone seeks to educate the public in small press publishing and encourage the growth of other small presses. Visit us online at www.starcherone.com and the Starcherone Superfan Group on Facebook. Starcherone Books, PO Box 303, Buffalo, NY 14201.

Starcherone Books is an independently operated imprint of Dzanc Books, distributed through Consortium Distribution and Small Press Distribution. We are a signatory to the Book Industry Treatise on Responsible Paper Use and use postconsumer recycled fiber paper in our books.